*The most accessible guide ever written to
the ancient practice of healing chants*

"You can use mantras to help you with any issue and to
change your life for the better," writes Thomas Ashley-
Farrand, an expert in Sanskrit mantras who has attracted a
loyal following through his lectures and Web site. Now, in
Healing Mantras, he has written a practical manual for
using mantras and the rhythms of healing sounds to help
solve everyday life and health problems.

Beginners will find here a lucid and solid grounding in
sound meditation, but even those who already practice
some energy-based techniques will discover much to
enrich their spiritual journey to healing and freedom.

Healing Mantras

USING SOUND AFFIRMATIONS
FOR PERSONAL POWER, CREATIVITY,
AND HEALING

THOMAS ASHLEY-FARRAND

Ballantine Wellspring ™

THE RANDOM HOUSE PUBLISHING GROUP • NEW YORK

A Ballantine Wellspring™ Book
Published by The Random House Publishing Group

Published in the United States by Ballantine Books, an imprint of The Random
House Publishing Group, a division of Random House, Inc., New York, and
simultaneously in Canada by Random House of Canada Limited, Toronto.

Ballantine is a registered trademark and Ballantine Wellspring™ and the Ballantine
Wellspring™ colophon are trademarks of Random House, Inc.

www.ballantinebooks.com

Library of Congress Cataloging-in-Publication Data
Ashley-Farrand, Thomas.
Healing mantras : using sound affirmations for personal power,
creativity, and healing / Thomas Ashley-Farrand.—1st ed.
p.   cm.
Includes bibliographical references and index.
ISBN 0-345-43170-7
1. Mantras.   I. Title.
BL560.A83   1999
291.3'7—dc21   99-12948

Cover design by Barbara Leff
Cover illustration by Vicki Rabinowicz
Text design by Ann Gold

Manufactured in the United States of America

First Edition: August 1999
22 24 26 28 29 27 25 23

In the beginning was the Word. And the Word was with God. And the Word was God. —John 1:1

On the spoken word all the Gods depend, all beasts and men; in the word live all creatures. . . . The word is the imperishable, the firstborn of eternal law, the mother of the Vedas, the navel of the divine world. —*Taittiriya Brahmana*

The speech of men cannot reach the Lords. . . . They must be addressed in their own language. . . . It is composed of sounds, not words. . . . This language, or the incantations of mantras being the most effective agent and the first of the keys which opens the door of communication between Mortals and Immortals. —H. P. Blavatsky, *The Secret Doctrine*

Contents

Acknowledgments

Many people have contributed to this work in direct and indirect ways. I want to acknowledge them here. First, I want to thank my agent, Stephany Evans of the Imprint Agency West, for her vision and confidence in this project right from the start. Her assistance has been invaluable throughout. I also want to thank literary agent Patricia Collins for her recommendation of my work to Stephany Evans.

Leslie Meredith, my editor at Ballantine Wellspring Books, has my gratitude for recognizing the value of this project immediately and framing a method for its fulfillment. She and her associate Cathy Elliott are performing a service of great value to authors and readers alike.

My thanks also goes to Stephany Evans and Mitch Sisskind for their help in the final preparation of the manuscript.

It is appropriate that I thank Michael and Wendy Weir for their constant unwavering support for this and other writing projects as they took shape. In the same spirit, I want to thank Dr. Doe Lang, author of *The Secrets of Charisma*, for her long-term and unflagging encouragement of my writing efforts.

Professor Marilyn Shaw, a true healer and wonderful teacher of healing, brought me to Chaffey College and introduced me to a group of students who are truly serious about learning and practicing various healing methods. I am grateful to her and to them.

Finally, last but first is my wife, Margalo Ashley-Farrand. It took her ten years of gentle persuasion to bring me to write my first book. For her support of and involvement in my writing projects, I am exceedingly grateful.

Healing
Mantras

Introduction: In the Beginning Was the Word

In spiritual and religious traditions all over the world, spiritual states are equated with light. A common spiritual objective is "enlightenment." In the everyday language of spiritual development, we seek "light on the path" so that we may safely make our way. For centuries, artists from diverse traditions have made use of light in depicting great spiritual teachers. A clear indicator of spiritual power, light surrounds the priests of the Ark of the Covenant and creates the nimbus of the saints, and halos of Christ and the Buddha. In the first few verses of Genesis we read, "And God said, *Let there be light, and there was light.*" Yet if we imagine that light is the highest expression of spiritual power, we are mistaken. The spirit is created and animated not by light, but by sound.

Looking more closely at Genesis we see, "God *said* . . ." The light of divine creation was initiated by sound. The *speech* of God, according to Genesis, was the source of the spiritual light to which we all aspire.

The New Testament Gospel of John, which was written thousands of years after Genesis, opens with the verse, "In the beginning was the *Word* . . ." The beginning was not light; rather, it was sound in the form of the divine speech. Neither the Old Testament nor the New Testament contains a verse such as "And God *made* light to shine." Rather, God creates the phenomenon by *speaking* of it. The primary mechanism of creation is sound.

3

In the wisdom of the ancient East, we find the same teaching. The whole universe comes about when God decides to manifest reality through the power of divine speech. In some Eastern texts, this power is referred to as Saraswati—the Word.

Sir John Woodroffe's *The Garland of Letters* includes a translation of a scripture called the *Sata patha Brahmana*, written many thousands of years ago. Volume 6 of that scripture opens:

> In the beginning was God with power through speech. God said, "May I be many . . . may I be propagated." And by his will expressed through subtle speech, he united himself with that speech and became pregnant. Prajapathi and Saraswati were then created. And Prajapathi is called the progenitor of all beings.

This statement sounds astonishingly similar to the idea of creation expressed in Genesis and the opening text of the Gospel of John.

A Brief Vedic Cosmology

Vedic religion, handed down for millennia through an oral tradition before the advent of writing, presents a concise summary of how the cosmos came about. Creation began with Being, a state so sublime and so different from anything we can conceive of that it can only be expressed in metaphors, allegories, and pictures. One of the most common representations of Being is the Hindu divinity Narayana, who floats in a sea of inky black. From the solar plexus of the sleeping Narayana springs another entity called Brahma.

As Narayana sleeps and Brahma is formed, the universe is conceived as a divine idea. Unmanifest, this universe is vague and unformed. But Being has moved to Mind, which is Brahma. This mind of Brahma, however, is not static but dynamic. It soon experiences Desire, which is quickly followed by Will. Desire and Will cause Brahma to call upon his power—Saraswati, the Divine Speech of manifestation. Saraswati is described as a feminine principle. She is "the Word" as understood in the Vedic tradition. When Brahma calls upon his power, when he calls upon Saraswati, the universe comes into being with all the forces that will animate it for billions of years to come.

The process of creation, then, is described through the images of a brief narrative:

> *First, God as Being . . .*
> *From Being comes Mind . . .*
> *From Mind comes Desire . . .*
> *From Desire comes Will . . .*
> *From Will comes the Word . . .*
> *From the Word comes everything else.*

Other Eastern texts express the same idea. Kuan Yin in Chinese Buddhism is referred to as "the divine voice," which calls forth the illusive form of the universe out of the seven elements. The Vedas speak of the divine sound-current Shabda Brahma, which permeates all and is a key to creation.

References in sacred texts to the power of sound are not limited to creation myths. In the Old Testament book of Exodus, the sound of trumpets is said to bring down the walls of Jericho. In the East, the trumpet sound is a symbol of great spiritual power associated with insight and elevated consciousness. The sound of the trumpet is thought to be "heard" or perceived through the third eye—a point between the eyebrows—which can have direct communication with the Divine.

More recent texts and teachers echo this ancient idea. Mystic Sufi master Hazrat Inayat Khan has written, "Divine sound is the cause of all manifestation. The knower of the mystery of sound knows the mystery of the whole universe." In the early part of the twentieth century, H. P. Blavatsky, founder of the Theosophical Society, wrote in *The Secret Doctrine*, "Sound is a tremendous occult [hidden] power. It is such a stupendous force that the electricity generated by a million Niagaras could never counteract even the smallest potentiality when directed by proper knowledge."

This last statement leads to the idea that the great power of sound that created the universe is also accessible to humanity. Scattered through various religious traditions, we find references to the divine power of words. The Latin word *cantare*, root of the English "cantor," is commonly translated as "to sing." However, some linguists believe that the original meaning was "to produce by magic." The Mexican Huichol Indians use the Spanish word *cantor*, "singer," to mean "shaman"—a clear indication of the power they attribute to the voice. Another Latin word, *carmen*, is often translated as "poem," but originally it meant "magic formula."*

Mystics' and Scientists' Views

Some scientists, too, have recognized the power of sound and sound waves, which are sometimes organized and expressed as music. The sixteenth-century astronomer Johannes Kepler wrote, "God was master of cosmic sound, causing the planets to leave their entirely circular orbits and to adopt consciously complicated elliptical orbits in order to produce ever more beautiful music." Kepler viewed the orbits of the planets as vibrations, the Music of the Spheres.

Some two thousand years earlier, the Greek mathematician and philosopher Pythagoras noted, "The seven heavens sounded each one vowel down to earth and became the creation of all things that be on earth." This statement could almost have come directly from a text of the Jewish mystical tradition known as the Kabbalah, in which the power of vowels is said to be divine. And the ancient rishis (sages) of India arrived at the same conclusion, teaching that the pronunciation of vowels corresponds to the vibration of the five inner planets:

*In *Nada Brahma: The World Is Sound*, by Joachim-Ernst Berendt.

O Venus
A Jupiter
E Saturn
I Mars
U Mercury

Ravi Shankar, the contemporary master of the classical music of India, refers to the sound of God's power as Nada Brahma, the divine sound that reverberates through the universe and the "subtle human body" we all carry with us. Shankar states, "Our tradition teaches us that sound is God. Music is a spiritual discipline that raises one's inner being to divine peacefulness and bliss. We are taught to work toward a fundamental goal of the knowledge of the unchanging and eternal essence of the universe. Our music reveals the essence of the universe it reflects. Through music, one can reach God." Elsewhere he writes, "Saint musicians such as Baiju Bavare, Swami Haridas or Mian Tan Sen performed miracles by performing certain *Ragas* [classical Indian compositions]. It is said that some could light fires or oil lamps by singing one raga, or bring rain, or melt stones, cause flowers to bloom, and attract ferocious wild animals to a peaceful quiet circle around their singing."

In Joachim-Ernst Berendt's *Nada Brahma: The World Is Sound*, astronomers Jeff Lightman and Robert M. Sickels describe fascinating sounds in their experiments with radio astronomy: "The edge of the galaxy becomes a noisy hissing cacophony of sound produced by quick shifts in molecular and atomic energy levels. . . . The giant planet Jupiter produces its own peculiar noise: huge rapid sighs like the intense roaring of a distant surge, triggered by Jovian electricity from storms of such intensity as to be worthy of the god whose name the planet bears. The sun makes noises too, hisses and crackling in quietude and roars of alarming intensity when it spews out giant portions of matter into space."

Rudolf Kippenhahn, director of the Max Planck Research Institute for Astrophysics in Munich, also wrote about the sound of the planets and objects of the heavens: "We hear the heterodyne ticking of pulsars . . . high energy pulses from spherical star clusters, with sequences which repeat themselves. In space, there is ticking, drumming, humming and crackling."

The great rhythms of the cosmos are also revealed through modern physics. In *The Silent Pulse*, George Leonard writes about the vastness of space that composes what we call matter: "We can see the fully crystalline structure of muscle fiber, waving like wheat in the wind, pulsing many trillions of times a second. . . . As we move closer to the nucleus, it begins to dissolve. It too is nothing more than an oscillating field [that] upon our approach dissolves into pure rhythm. . . . Of what is the body made? It is made of emptiness and rhythm. At the heart of the world, there is no solidarity, there is only dance."

The power of sound, the power of music, the power of vowels, and the power of speech are the great creative forces of the universe: as custodians of these, human beings possess tremendous spiritual power. For centuries, mystical scriptures and teachers of the East have taught mantra as a means for harnessing this power.

The Mantra Toolbox

Mantra is a Sanskrit word with many shades of meaning: "tool of the mind," "divine speech," and "language of the human spiritual physiology" are just a few of these. In the context of this book, mantra is a tool for healing problems that we all face in life. As the mystic Sufi master Vilayat Inayat Khan states, "The practice of mantra actually kneads the flesh of the body with sound. The delicate cells of the elaborate bundles of nerves are subjected to a constant hammering, a seizure of the flesh by the vibrations of divine sound."

Mantra can help you feel more peaceful or more energized. It can help you cope with illness and it can sometimes help effect physical healing. It can help you deal with difficult or unpleasant circumstances, by helping you to see a course of action, or it can give you the patience and perspective to just "wait it out." It can help you bring your wishes to fruition and create reality from your dreams. Mantra is a dynamic, individual, nonviolent way to approach conditions you wish to change. They are ancient formulas of divine sounds recorded by the ancient sages of India and held in trust and in secret for ages in both India and Tibet.

But mantra is not a panacea. It is not usually the only way or even the best way to solve human problems. Your life and your karma—the accumulated effect of all your thoughts and actions over many lives—are far too complex to be completely mastered by several weeks of work with spiritual formulas, no matter how powerful they might be. But mantra can completely solve many of the problems we face, and it can considerably soften others.

Life and Desires

Mantra can help you deal with the material concerns and necessities of life. All of us want or need something, or wish to make changes in our lives. Some of us want a mate. Others desire a new job or career. Many of us have faced health problems or know someone who has. People struggle with financial woes and the many life transitions. We have desires that can be as simple as a new car or as complicated as smoothing out some tangled family mess.

Many of us also want help in managing our emotions and inner lives. We encounter situations that produce knee-jerk reactions that we would like to prevent. We become frustrated, sad, angry, jealous. Sometimes our responses can be more problematic than the situations that caused them. A few words spoken in anger can do harm on a grand scale to a friendship or love relationship. Depression can become so severe that it drives everyone and everything from us. Longings and obsessions isolate us. Mantra practice can help you gain clarity about your life, your purpose, and yourself.

Sometimes we would just like to be able to help others, but we may not know exactly how to help. A family member or coworker may be in some difficulty, or we would like to be able to make a contribution to the good of our neighborhood or the world—if only we knew what to do. Mantra can help you find the right course of action for effective change.

The relatively simple tool of mantra can help you with all the conditions and challenges you need to face. Even though mantra is ancient in origin, you can apply it to virtually any contemporary issue with good results.

The Mantra Stockpiles

Modern scholars and Vedic priests differ about the age of mantra writings. Some scholars date the earliest written records of the four Vedic scriptures to 1000 B.C.E., although the oldest written version of the Rig Veda in existence dates from only the fourteenth century C.E. Yet in *The Principal Upanishads*, the respected scholar S. Radhakrishnan, quoting from Bloomfield's *The Religion of the Vedas*, states, "The Vedas are not only the most ancient literary monument of India, but also the most ancient literature of the Indo-European peoples, earlier than that of Greece or Israel."* The earliest hymns and mantras contained in the Rig Veda are traditionally considered to date back to 1500 B.C.E. and possibly even to before 4000 B.C.E.

Hindu priests emphatically assert that mantra writings are much older than academic authorities believe. The popularly accepted history of mantra, which even today is conveyed through an oral tradition taught in Hindu temples, places the earliest writing at the time of the *Mahabharata*, some three thousand years before Christ. And Sanskrit mantras existed at least two thousand years *before that* in myth, story, and legend.

The Vedic teachings were originally reserved for the priest class,

---

*Although Bloomfield's *Religion of the Vedas* (published in 1908) is referred to three times over the course of this massive 950-page book, his first name and other publishing information are not provided.

and its rituals, as well as the Vedas themselves and the mantras contained within them, were transmitted orally for thousands of years. After passing orally from generation to generation, Sanskrit mantras were first written on palm leaves so that they could be preserved. The first "librarians" were families who dedicated themselves to preserving these mantra writings. Cataloged by subject, application, and outcome, the mantras were meticulously stored and sheltered from the elements. When the palm leaves became brittle or moldy, the mantras were recopied onto fresh leaves while they were still legible.

As the stockpile of mantras became larger and larger, even whole families could not keep up with the recopying needed to maintain the library. For keeping abreast of the ever-accumulating new mantra information, summaries of some sections were created. These summaries condensed whole shelves of subject material down to a handful of leaves. This worked for several centuries until the stockpile again grew too large. Then the contents were summarized again. More hundreds and hundreds of years passed until the whole cycle was repeated once again. Throughout the several thousand years during which the summaries were being compiled, certain sections were considered so important that they were never summarized, but remained intact.

These Hindu teachings of inspiration and insight followed a similar path from oral transmission to transcription in Sanskrit. The Upanishads are the summaries of the summaries of the summaries of teachings created many thousands of years ago. The Upanishads contain the Forest Cantos, or Aranyakas, and the Brahmanas, which are fragments of larger, lost works. The four Vedas survived nearly untouched and unsummarized: Rig Veda, Artharva Veda, Yajur Veda, and Sama Veda. In a sense, the Vedas and the Upanishads are all collections of Sanskrit mantras linked together and intended to convey timeless ideas on a wide range of subjects.

The amount of information contained even in these fragmented summaries is staggering. A whole system of medicine is contained in the Artharva Veda—a system that Western medicine has only recently begun to acknowledge as valid. In the Rig Veda, spiritual matters of cosmology and individual development are set forth in grand mystical phrases and practices. Between 1000 B.C.E. and the end of the first Christian millennium, sages, scholars, and mystics such as Patañjali (200 B.C.E.), Shankaracharya (800 A.D.), and others presented even more specific practices for spiritual development and solutions to problems. It is from these teachings that Sanskrit acquired the title Deva Lingua, or "language of the gods," which connotes that even mortals can commune with the gods and become like them: powerful and immortal. The first requirement, however, is to learn to "speak the language" and thereby use the power it contains. Mantra is the language through which we invoke the gods and their energy.

Deva Lingua

While mantras, the Vedas, and the Upanishads are all written in Sanskrit, this language is no longer spoken in everyday conversation. Because Sanskrit is not spoken widely among the general population of any country, it is technically classified a "dead" language. Yet all Hindu religious practices and traditions are taught, conducted, and transmitted in Sanskrit. Most Buddhist practices that use the spoken word still contain the bulk of their material in Sanskrit. All of the swamis and teachers from India who have come to the West use systems of personal development derived from Sanskrit texts. So, to call Sanskrit a dead language does not take into account the daily practices of many millions of people.

Moreover, many Western languages can trace their roots to Sanskrit, which dictionaries often classify as Indo-European. Sanskrit truly deserves its other title, the Mother of Tongues, as scholars describe it. In Sanskrit, *mata* is "mother" and *pitra* is "father"; these are obviously close to the Latin *mater* and *pater*. The Romance languages (Spanish, Italian, Portuguese, French, and Romanian) derive from Latin, which is itself derived from Sanskrit, which was spoken for many centuries before Latin came into existence.

The Experiment

Over the years, I have learned many mantras for solving life's problems. To give you some idea of how this can work, I'd like to tell you how a mantra helped me through a particularly difficult time.

In 1980, many things changed for me. For eight years, I had been priest-in-residence at a spiritual center affiliated with a group in India, but based in Washington, D.C. I enjoyed being of service, and my responsibilities by and large were pleasant. However, the conduct of the organization's Indian leader was making me more and more uncomfortable, because he was behaving inappropriately regarding issues of sex, money, and power. I vacillated between staying and leaving, and the worry was enervating.

One day, in one of my usual two-hour meditation sessions, I saw a clock that read a quarter to twelve. I was shown that at twelve o'clock, the relationship I had long been seeking would arrive. I resolved to wait awhile before coming to a decision about leaving the center. As it turned out, those fifteen minutes took more than six months in real-world time. After six months, a woman named Margalo arrived at the organization. Within two weeks, I had left the center to move in with her. One year later we were married, and we decided to leave the organization altogether.

When I had first become involved with the organization, I was working as a television producer. Fairly soon after joining, I had become a full-time instructor in broadcasting at George Washington University. In 1980, however, my non-tenure-track contract was up and, newly married, I was considering my professional options. Margalo suggested we leave Washington, D.C., for her former home in southern California. I saw no reason to refuse. Once there, I knew I would have to develop a new career for myself. But despite all my efforts to find a job in Los Angeles, the media capital of the Western world, doors in broadcasting remained closed, and I was forced to take temporary jobs. I struggled to create some kind of balance between my discouraging search for a profession and my new, happy life with my wife.

During my years as a priest, I had used Sanskrit mantras almost exclusively in meditations to strengthen my focus and to foster spiritual insights. For any secular problem, I would return to prayers that I had learned from my Judeo-Christian upbringing in the Presbyterian and Methodist churches. Using mantras does not mean you have to leave your present religious organization or your roots or abandon other spiritual practices. While I still consider myself a Christian, I have explored many religious traditions, and over the years I have added other spiritual observances of Hindu and Buddhist origins to my daily practices to form a personal spirituality and practice of compassion and service. Mantra is a wonderfully effective complementary spiritual practice that can enrich your life.

In any case, the results I had obtained from prayers were sporadic, but I had accepted them. At this low point in my professional life, however, I decided to apply a mantra to my situation to see if it would help me. I chose a mantra that seemed appropriate for my difficulties in the material world, and I decided to work with it for forty days. I chose a forty-day practice because forty is a recurrent number in religious literature. Jesus went into the wilderness for forty days. Noah tossed upon the seas for forty days. Moses wandered through the desert for forty years. The Buddha provided a variation by sitting under the Bodhi Tree for forty-three days until he achieved enlightenment. In Vedic Hinduism, forty days is the standard length for a concentrated mantra discipline. In Roman Catholicism, the novena, a daily discipline of prayer employed by the faithful to seek help in solving life's problems, is sometimes observed for five days, forty days, and fifty-four days, although it is traditionally done for nine days.

I figured that I needed a significant amount of time for my mantra practice to influence whatever forces were preventing me from finding a job. The intention I formed in my mind was to find a steady job in which I could make a contribution to others, and from which I could receive a living wage. Since many problem-solving mantras are general in nature, the mantra I selected was one for removal of obstacles:

Om Gum Ganapatayei Namaha

(OM GUM GUH-NUH-PUH-TUH-YEI NAHM-AH-HA)

"Om and salutations to the remover of obstacles
for which Gum is the seed."

Among Vedic and Hindu sects, this mantra (which will be discussed in chapter 5) is universally acknowledged as supremely effective for clearing away obstacles of all sorts. Since I did not know what was preventing me from finding steady, gainful employment, my goal was to remove any obstacle, internal or external, spiritual or physical, standing between me and the right kind of job.

For the next forty days, I repeated the mantra as much as I could, sometimes silently, sometimes out loud. While performing household chores, I would chant the mantra. While driving, I would chant it in my car. While eating or preparing food, I chanted it. When falling off into sleep I would keep the mantra going as long as I could. Upon waking, I would immediately begin chanting the mantra. If I was with other people, I would chant silently. If I was alone, I would chant softly out loud. I became an *Om Gum Ganapatayei Namaha* chanting machine.

I liked the way the mantra made me feel. The rhythm of it quickly settled into my consciousness, and I found that after two weeks the mantra would start by itself if I was otherwise engaged. Waking up in the middle of the night, I could hear it faintly going on in some rear compartment of my mind. It agreed with my body and mind as if it were a nutritious, spiritual food.

After three weeks of working with the mantra, I was called upon to perform a Vedic ceremony for a group in Santa Ana. The ceremony lasted about an hour, and when it was over I circulated among the guests to chat and munch on snacks. With one small group, the conversation eventually got around to "And what do you do for a living?" I somewhat awkwardly explained that I was new to the West Coast and had not settled into any one thing yet.

After further conversation, one of the women in the group said that her company was looking for someone to help with a marketing project for the next three months. I inquired about the kind of work they did and she replied that it was a medical care facility that performed family practice, occupational medicine, and urgent care. I knew nothing about the health care field and said so.

Undeterred, the woman pressed me to call her and schedule an appointment for the next week. I assented, mostly out of courtesy and a sense that I should explore every possibility—but without any real hope of finding employment.

When I arrived for my appointment, I was met by my acquaintance's boss, Rick, who interviewed me for about ten minutes. I believed I was sunk because I showed no real understanding of their industry, but much to my surprise he finished his short interview with, "I think you will work out just fine. But I need to get the docs to sign off on it. Please wait here."

The doctors approved me and within minutes I had filled out some paperwork and become their clinic marketing representative performing fieldwork on a three-month temporary assignment. The pay was modest, but it beat temporary work or waiting by the phone, so I was grateful. All the while, I kept chanting the mantra silently inside.

After several days of making business calls, I learned enough to realize that the marketing materials I had to support my calls were just terrible. I couldn't banish this realization from my mind, and I began to feel more and more foolish as I made the calls. Finally, I had to do something.

At this point, I was on day thirty of my forty-day chanting discipline. That night, I reworked everything into three new pieces, using the colors of the building and the familiar caduceus medical symbol. When I arrived at the office the next morning, I sought out the doctor to whom I reported and briefly showed him what I had in mind. He stopped dead, looked at me, and said to meet him in the conference room in one hour. When I entered the conference room there was Rick, along with the woman who had suggested I apply for the job, the doctor who had interviewed me, and two other doctors who were partners at the facility. Unsettled, I realized that I was about to give a presentation. The doctor who had called the meeting said, "Show us what you've got."

After my ten-minute impromptu presentation, the docs asked me to leave the room for a few minutes. I nervously complied. When I was asked back in, my boss said, "Congratulations, you're our new marketing director. Get yourself some cards printed and also get this new stuff you designed printed as soon as possible." I was in shock, but still going on inside was *Om Gum Ganapatayei Namaha.*

I finished out my forty-day mantra discipline without further incident. Within the next thirty days I was involved in a joint marketing project with a local hospital. The nurse who was the hospital's marketing director was friendly and technically very skilled. We worked well together. When we were nearly finished with the project, she asked if I would mind telling what they paid me. I did not mind, and told her. She wrinkled up her face and said, "They're getting you cheap."

After the joint project was finished, my boss congratulated us both on a job well done. After shaking his hand, the nurse motioned toward me and said, "You know this guy is wa-a-a-a-y underpaid. You better be careful or someone will make him an offer and he'll get away from you." I was flabbergasted, but my boss responded like a pro in every way. He grinned and said, "Don't you worry, we'll take good care of him." Within thirty days I had a 40 percent raise.

That was early in 1983. I stayed with this company for nearly seven years. I had numerous raises and felt I was appreciated for my work. I finally left when my supervisor decided to form his own company and made me an offer to join him.

I attributed my successful job search to my mantra discipline. Its effectiveness made a huge impression upon me, and I had a new appreciation for the power of spiritual formulas in solving everyday difficulties. I began to recommend mantras to others for their problems and they worked amazingly well.

I gave this same mantra to a friend of mine in Washington, D.C., who had just retired from a career in the Army. He had studied gemology and desired to find a job in that field. After searching for months in many cities, however, he was unable to find the work he wanted. I recommended that he begin chanting *Om Gum Ganapatayei Namaha* as much as he could for ten days. On the eleventh day, I performed an energy-cleansing ceremony on his behalf. Within three days he had several job offers and was well-started on his new career.

As another example of how mantras can be used to help us cope with problems in our daily lives, a friend of mine, Rae, was bothered by terrible neighbors across the street and next door. Those across the street would intentionally park in front of her house, blocking her driveway and making it impossible for her to get out, or for the trash haulers to pick up her garbage. Although she had called the police, they could only help her from time to time. The neighbors next to her were constantly noisy and resisted any request for consideration. Rae asked for my help and I gave her this mantra:

Narasimha Ta Va Da So Hum

(NAH-RAH-SEEM-HA TAH VAH DAH SOH HOOM)

Narasimha invokes the energy for destroying the seemingly indestructible. *Ta, Va,* and *Da* invoke energies of the body and direct the energy the mantra creates to accomplish the highest good. *So Hum* is a mantra unto itself; it puts the mind in tune with the divine self within.

Rae began to chant this mantra many times every day. She quickly grew fond of the mantra, which felt good to her, and it helped her feel strong and positive in the face of her neighbors' disruptions. After about two months, her noisy neighbors sold their house and moved away. As of this writing, the neighbors across the street are gone a good deal of the time and the problem with them has lessened considerably.

This mantra is also helping her build inner strength for her career in service to others.

Chanting a Sanskrit mantra alone did not land me my job with the medical clinic, but it helped me approach new possibilities and a new career with positive expectations. I believe that our mantras also helped my friends and me to maintain a calm and peaceful state of mind and body so that we were receptive to insights about how best to work through the challenges that presented themselves. Mantra practice also provided me with the energy and concentration to accomplish what I needed to do, and the inner confidence to make a worthwhile contribution in a field about which I had previously known nothing. It was the catalyst for a cascade of positive transformations and developments in my and my friends' lives.

In *Healing Mantras*, I catalog the success of my students and friends in their use of mantras. The book is intended to provide you with a toolbox of mantras to correct and heal various conditions in your life. These spiritual formulas can also help you create abundance, unlock creative power within you, and aid in manifesting a fuller life in every way. It is my prayer that you will succeed beyond all your expectations.

1

Sound, Music, and Healing

L isten . . .
   Listen closely . . .
      What sounds can you hear right now? Chances are, there are
many of them. Our lives are filled with sounds of all kinds, and our responses to those sounds help create who we are from moment to moment and from year to year. At one extreme irritating or annoying, at
the other pleasant or deeply satisfying, sound vibrations affect our
thoughts, our feelings, and how we experience the world.

A quiet moment of concentration quickly evaporates when a
diesel backhoe starts tearing up the street outside your house. At the
whine of a gasoline-powered leaf blower, a normally placid person
turns into a red-eyed monster seeking revenge. Loud music playing,
dogs barking, babies crying—they can all be very disconcerting, especially if they belong to someone else!

Yet a few whispered phrases from a lover can instantly transform
sadness into euphoria. The cooing of a baby gazing trustingly into our
eyes produces joy that melts all care. Tensions dissolve when we hear
some bars from a Mozart concerto. All this because of a few vibrations.

Sound can change our entire life's course in an instant. Words
spoken in anger can cause permanent problems between a husband
and wife, or parent and child. The throb of a well-tuned motor can en-
gender such satisfaction in an amateur mechanic that a whole new career path suddenly opens before him. A word of encouragement from a

teacher at just the right time can inspire a student for many years
to come.

We respond to all these sounds, but usually we don't give them
much conscious attention. We don't really think about them. They influence us, but we go on largely unaware that we have been touched
by an ancient wisdom . . . a force of nature . . . an instrument of God.

Ancient Greece: Pythagoras and Healing Sound

Throughout history, the power of sound has been recognized, celebrated, and investigated. The Greek philosopher Pythagoras, who developed basic principles in mathematics and astronomy, was also one
of the earliest investigators of the physical, emotional, and spiritual
effects of sound. His sophisticated descriptions of vibration and har-
monics anticipated modern research to an amazing degree. Using
vibrating strings, the philosopher with his students worked out the
mathematical relationships between sounds, and he proposed, in his
doctrine of the harmony of spheres, that the ratios between musical
notes were also expressed in the distances between Earth and the
other planets.

One of the cornerstones of Pythagorean philosophy is the idea
that beauty and proportion—qualities commonly found in mathematics, nature, and especially music—are transferable to the observer.
Just as a plucked string can cause another string to vibrate, we can begin to resonate in harmony with natural beauty by studying and appre-
ciating it. By exposing ourselves to the wonders of nature, we can
foster an internal harmony that benefits every aspect of our being.

In the several schools of philosophy guided by Pythagoras in
Greece and Italy, music was actually used as a kind of spiritual medicine. Certain melodies and instruments were prescribed for anger,
sadness, and other so-called passions of the mind. At the end of each

day, Pythagoreans were instructed to achieve serenity by listening to certain poems and musical compositions.

All this has obvious similarities to the use of healing mantras. Both the musical compositions recommended by Pythagoras and the mantras presented in these pages are intended to deal with specific problems and aspirations. Both use combinations of sound to eliminate inner dissonance and nurture harmony. For both Pythagoras and the tradition of Sanskrit mantras, sound is more than simply a medium of artistic expression. Sound has practical and powerful applications in the real world. Sound can help, and sound can heal.

The Renaissance and the Power of Poetry

During the sixteenth century, when Elizabeth I ruled England, the most learned man in the realm was a Cambridge-educated scholar named John Dee. Not simply an academic, Dee was a student of the mystical arts of alchemy and astrology, and he had a profound interest in the effects of music, rhythm, and the spoken word on human consciousness. Dee believed, as did some of the most gifted poets of his time both in England and on the Continent, that sound could be used to heal the most intense political antagonisms of their time.

Throughout Elizabeth's reign, there was a constant threat of war between Protestant Britain and the Catholic powers of France and Spain. As one of the queen's personal confidants, Dee was intensely interested in pacifying this dangerous situation. The solution he came up with seems incredible by today's standards, but it must be understood in the context of a period in which language and music were still associated with incantations, spells, and the conjuring of spirits. Poetry, which was almost always recited or sung to musical accompaniment, was not just an artistic diversion. Like prayer, it was considered by Dee and his circle to be a way of invoking magical powers.

If the proper words were associated with the appropriate music, Dee believed, a purifying effect would occur in the minds and hearts of listeners, and political and religious hatreds would be put aside. He found a mythological basis for this idea in the Greek legend of Orpheus, who entered the land of the dead and returned safely because of his hypnotic musical talents. The biblical story of David provided another model. If David's lute music could calm the spirit of the mad King Saul, as the Bible said, perhaps there was reason to believe that sound could indeed bring peace to the known world.

Working in secret with a cabal of aristocratic poets in both England and France, John Dee developed measured poetic rhythms that were intended to bring about world peace. Think of it: This was a top-secret project undertaken by some of the most learned and prominent men of their time—and it was intended to prevent international conflict simply through music and the spoken word.

Although Dee's poetic experiments did not prevent the attack of the Spanish armada or the bloody religious conflicts that continued throughout Elizabeth's reign, it illustrates the power ascribed to sound and speech during the most glorious period of the English Renaissance. This view of sound's political capabilities was not limited to that time. Two centuries later, Napoleon declared that the revolutionary anthem known as the "Marseillaise" was more valuable than two regiments of troops. It's impossible to imagine the civil rights movement of the 1960s without "We Shall Overcome." Every war has been accompanied by music, with military instruments and motivating hymns to inspire the fighting forces and people on the home front. As the magician John Dee realized, sound has the power to transform people's lives, and even to change the world.

Indeed, human cultures have used sound for centuries in the peaceful healing and transformation of ailments and conditions of all kinds. As Ted Andrews writes in *Music Therapy for Non-Musicians*, "Chinese healers [have] used singing stones—thin flat pieces of jade which emit various musical tones when struck or played like a xylophone. The Sufis consider *Hu* to be the ultimate creative sound, chanting and singing it to create changes in consciousness. Tibetans consider *Kung* to be the great tone of nature. . . . Shamans in many aboriginal and native societies use drums, rattles and flutes [and chants, as we shall later see] to heal the body and touch other realms. . . . Every aspect of sound was recognized for its ability to effect changes in body, mind and spirit."

My Petunias Love Your Band

Music's well-documented effects extend even to other life forms. In his book *The Secret Life of Plants*, Peter Tompkins describes an experiment in which four plant groups were given identical lighting, soil, watering schedule, and so forth. One group listened to rock and roll for several hours each day. A second group heard jazz, and a third, classical compositions. The remaining plants formed a control group that had no musical stimulus whatsoever.

Within a few days, the plants exposed to rock and roll had inclined away from the speakers at a thirty-degree angle. They were also somewhat stunted in their growth compared to the control group. The plants exposed to jazz exhibited various results, depending upon the artist; they seemed particularly fond of Duke Ellington and Louis Armstrong. But the most dramatic results were seen in the plants that heard classical music. They had grown more than any other group. What's more, they had aligned themselves at a sixty-degree angle toward the speakers, as if trying to get as close to the source of the sound as possible. A "favorite" sound of these plants were recordings of Ravi Shankar playing ragas—the Indian equivalent of Western symphonies.

This procedure has been repeated, with similar results. In 1970, a version of the experiment performed by some college students was reported on the *CBS Evening News*. One of the students had shown the results on videotape to a local rock musician and received this startled response: "If rock music does that to the plants, what's it doing to me?"

During the last decade, other research on the beneficial physical and psychological effects of music has yielded the following:

"Students who study music scored higher on both the verbal and math portions of the SAT than nonmusic students."
—College Entrance Examination Board, October 1996

"In a study of medical school applicants, 66 percent of music majors who applied to medical school were admitted, the highest percentage of any group. Only 44 percent of biochemistry majors were admitted."
—Lewis Thomas, Phi Beta Kappa lecture, February 1994

"At-risk children who participated in an arts program that included music showed significant increases in overall self-concept."
—N. H. Berry, Auburn University, 1992

"Preschoolers who studied piano performed 34 percent better in spatial and temporal reasoning ability than preschoolers who spent the same amount of time learning to use computers."
—F. H. Rauscher and G. L. Shaw, *Neurological Research,* February 1997

"Listening to music can increase levels of interleukin-1 (IL-1) in the blood from 12.5 percent to 14 percent. Interleukins are a family of proteins associated with blood and platelet production, lymphocyte stimulation and cellular protection against AIDS, cancer and other diseases." —Michigan State University, reported in Don Campbell, *The Mozart Effect**

The chanting of songs, verses, and mystic formulas existed long before the development of even the most primitive instruments. In modern times, the healing benefits of liturgical chanting have only recently been rediscovered, and in an interesting way.

During the 1960s there was a very clear instance of sound's potential to affect human health. For centuries the monks of a certain

*Source: www.mozarteffect.com

Benedictine monastery in France had chanted several hours every day. Then, during the 1960s, the Second Vatican Council began considering alterations in church practices, including changing the language of chant from the traditional Latin to languages spoken locally. But when the Council could not agree on the language issue, it was decided instead to end chanting altogether and replace it with other, more productive activities.

When this new routine went into effect, the Benedictine monks began to change. For hundreds of years the order had thrived on only three or four hours of sleep, but now the monks became listless and fatigued. Even when their schedule was further altered to allow more sleep, they were constantly weary. A change in diet was implemented. A seven-hundred-year tradition of vegetarianism was replaced by a diet that included meat, but the monks' health did not improve.

Then Dr. Alfred Tomatis, an ear specialist, visited the monastery and tested the monks' hearing. Many of them turned out to be hearing-impaired, though the cause was unclear. The only variable seemed to be the cessation of chanting. Dr. Tomatis recommended that chanting resume. After the monks returned to their old routine, a transformation very quickly took place among them. Most of them again became able to function with minimal sleep.

Dr. Tomatis later told this story to a Canadian broadcast audience and explained that the cerebral cortex can become "charged," or positively stimulated, by certain kinds and frequencies of sound. Through their daily chanting sessions, the Benedictines were bringing energy into their bodies and their minds.

Indigenous Traditions of Chanting and Mantras

The chanting human voice, in fact, is the world's oldest musical instrument. Every culture and civilization has recognized its magical power. Chant traditions span the centuries and are steeped in ritual and sacred ceremony. There are chants for praising the gods and goddesses of every religion, and invoking healing for a multitude of afflictions and illnesses. At certain times and in certain places, these traditions have been practiced only by an elite group of priests or initiates. To this day, many chants remain unknown to the world at large.

Aborigines.

The indigenous peoples of Australia, for instance, allow only a certain number of their chants to be heard by outsiders. One of those visitors was the British anthropologist A. P. Elkin. In *The Australian Aborigines*, Elkin reported hearing "Byzantine-like solemn chanting in iambic measures by male voices in unison to Kunapipi, the Mother Goddess cult of the Central North. . . . It can best be likened to the chanting of the ritual psalms in the Book of Common Prayer."

In the rituals of the Aborigine medicine men and sorcerers, chant seems to serve the purpose of navigating a complex system of taboos and inflicting harm upon enemies. But as Elkin pointed out, "We know very little about these practices. Great secrecy is attached to what is chanted. Moreover, some chants include words of deep secret significance."

The Mbuti.

In other parts of the world, indigenous peoples are more willing to share their secrets with outsiders. Some years ago, as I stood in a long check-cashing line at George Washington University, I recognized the world-renowned anthropologist Colin Turnbull standing behind me. I knew of Turnbull's travels in Africa and suspected that he was familiar with African chanting rituals. So I struck up a conversation, expressing my interest in chanting, in particular the traditions of India and Tibet. Turnbull said that he had spent time in both places, and then tested me a bit by asking me to chant a series of Tibetan mantras, and then some Shakti mantras from India. I apparently passed his inspection, because for the next several minutes we shared an extraordinary conversation.

Turnbull had spent two years in central Africa living among the Mbuti Pygmies, who let him in on the secrets of their chant to the forest, which they called the *molimo*. According to Turnbull, the Mbuti had an extensive store of practical wisdom. They could cure headaches and stomachaches, they had herbs to relieve fevers, and they knew how to set broken limbs. But their principal method of healing and problem solving involved chanting to the forest for help.

"The Mbuti would chant most of the night," Turnbull told me. "This could go on for as long as a month, and during the whole time no one got more than a few hours' sleep per night."

"But how were the problems solved by chanting to the forest?" I asked.

"Well," he said, drawing his lanky frame full upright and clearly enjoying himself, "by the end of the chant the problem just didn't seem to exist anymore. It just sort of went away."

Later I found more detailed information on the Mbuti in Turnbull's books. In *Wayward Servants*, he writes, "All chants share the same essential nature, share the same power of sound. The sound 'awakens' the forest in Mbuti terminology, and the nature of the sound indicates the particular area of interest of the Mbuti at the moment, thus attracting the forest's attention to the immediate needs of its children. It is also the essential nature of all chants that they should be pleasing to the forest. . . . The Mbuti are accustomed to waiting for situations to improve. If bad hunting persists, or sickness shows no sign of abating, then it becomes a matter of the forest." In the evenings, the men gather around a central fire and sing *molimo* songs.

The Mbuti believe that all they have to do is awaken the forest, which is by nature benevolent, and their problem will be solved. Interestingly, even though all life as they know it depends upon the forest, Turnbull tells us, "the Mbuti believe that man himself is, in part, spiritual and that his life derives not from the flesh [or forest] but from some other source."

That day in the check-cashing line, Turnbull told me that he had wanted to do something quite different with his life. As a boy of sixteen, he had journeyed to Tibet. He went to a certain temple every day, and there he grew to love the sonorous resonance that is so uniquely characteristic of Tibetan chanting. One day, he happened upon a woman monk there, instructing some younger monks who were about Turnbull's age. Without understanding any of what was being said, Turnbull went back every day to hear her instructions and the chants that were always part of her teachings.

After several days, the monk acknowledged him and through an interpreter asked what he wanted. Young Turnbull replied that he wanted to remain there and study with her. Looking vaguely off into the sky, she seemed to go away for a few moments. Then, returning her gaze to him, she declared that staying in Tibet was not Colin Turnbull's dharma—his life's purpose or path—in this incarnation. Instead, he was to travel around the world, live in many places, and write books.

Turnbull told me he had cried like a baby at those words. Yet his life turned out exactly as she had said. His initial attraction to chant followed him for the rest of his life, as he lived among many cultures and experienced their chanting rituals.

The Melanesians.
The Melanesian traders of New Guinea are the world's most practical and focused practitioners of chant. Their lives are regulated by a complex code of procedures known as the *kula*, to which all chanting practices are related. Rituals and chants enable the Melanesians to move from place to place, obtain the best price for their goods, appease dangerous water spirits, and ensure that they catch the right fish at the right time. All chanting is related to the *kula* and to achieving optimum results in the practical activities of everyday life.

Stories are told of the most effective magicians and chanters. As I read *Argonauts of the Western Pacific*, Bronislaw Malinowski's fascinating account of his experiences among the Papuans of Melanesian New Guinea, I recognized intriguing parallels with Vedic knowledge and practice. For instance, a legendary Melanesian priest was named Omkarana—and in Sanskrit, the Omkara is the sound-name for the sacred syllable *Om*, which has become familiar in the West. Someone who has achieved Omkara is at a high spiritual state and would qualify as a high priest.

In Melanesian legend, the mythical sorcerer is always accompanied by a dog. In India, back in the mists of early Vedic Hinduism, the very first guru is described as a young boy named Dattatreya who was always accompanied by a dog. He was called the greatest magician of his time. A practitioner of sorcery is a *geru* in the Melanesian language, just as the Sanskrit word *guru* means an enlightened spiritual teacher.

Mythical flying vehicles used in everyday activities are found in both Papuan and Vedic lore. Native oral history of New Guinea is peppered with references to flying canoes. The Indian epic known as the *Ramayana* includes descriptions of flying horse carriages.

The Melanesians, according to Malinowski, believe that "all magic comes from the netherworld." Magic does not derive from dreams, nor was it bestowed by the spirits who gave songs and dances to humanity. Rather, magic comes from its own place in the netherworld. Its power depends on specific magical formulas and the nature of individuals who utter them. And those are the very same conditions that apply to the use of Sanskrit mantras.

Native Americans.
Chant plays a special role in Native American spirituality. The Cibecue Apaches of Northeastern Arizona, for example, retain close ties to the old traditions. Dozens of sacred ceremonies are performed each year for healing and problem solving, and there is an intricate system of "powers" that can be used by medicine men and common people alike. These powers may be called upon at any time, whether in a life-or-death crisis or the activities of daily life.

At least twenty-eight different powers have been identified. Each power is connected to a specific animal and reflects that animal's actual or mythological qualities. Bat power, for example, makes possible undetected escapes from difficult circumstances. White-tailed deer power, bear power, coyote power, owl power, and many more, all have practical value in daily life. You gain access to a power by using appropriate chants and songs.

There are up to fifty-five chants for each power, with each chant containing as many as twenty-six verses. Chants must be sung in a carefully designated sequence, and hundreds of variations must be learned in order to gather a particular power to oneself.

Powers can be acquired in two ways. Rarely, a power simply "comes to a person." Acquiring a power from a medicine man is more usual, but still not a common practice due to the expense. A fee must be paid to the medicine man, and he must be supported for as long as it takes to learn the chants, which may be several months. Medicine men are usually born to the job, and they acquire the chants in childhood, but anyone who can pay is qualified to learn the chants of a particular power.

Tough economic times have thinned the ranks of the Apache medicine men, but there are still people who want a power and who can afford both the price and the time. In *The Cibecue Apache*, Keith Basso recorded comments from ordinary Apaches about how their power had helped them in daily life:

> "I use it on horses mostly. Sometimes they get wild and don't want to let you ride them. I use it then to make them gentle. In the mornings, sometimes, I can't find my horses. They wander off. It tells me where they are and I can go and find them."

> "The one I know, I use it for a lot of things. Deer hunting sometimes. It can tell me when to go and take me to a place where it is easy to kill one. Easy places, where it isn't hard to pack the meat out."

> "It's gone now, but I had it one time. It just watched out for me mostly. Once when they played *se* [a native gambling game] over at Oak Creek, I was sure far behind. Then I went away from where they were playing and prayed to it. When I came back, I started to win. My power made it that way."

> "I tell it to keep my kids from getting sick. Before I got it, our first baby died. Just overnight. Then I got it. We had six children and they don't get sick. It knows what I want to do is good, so it does it."

As complicated as the Apache chanting rituals are, those of the Navajo are reputed to be even more complex. In both cultures, the chanting rituals cover healing of illnesses as well as problems in daily living. In this regard, they have much in common with the mantra chanting from Vedic Hinduism.

I had my own experience with Native American chanting when a friend introduced me to Chief Joseph, a Native American leader who was also called Beautiful Painted Arrow by some of his followers. A meeting between us was arranged when he visited Los Angeles. Observing tradition, I brought a gift of tobacco, and when I made the presentation he asked if he could chant the blessing of the eagle feather for me. I replied that it would be my pleasure to receive it, and that I would then like to chant for him the blessing of Vishnu, the mantra protection brighter than a thousand suns. Chief Joseph loved the idea.

Holding a huge eagle feather over my head, he chanted for two or three minutes in a melodious yet powerful singsong manner. All the time he waved the eagle feather as if it were flying. I could feel not only the movement of air caused by the feather, but also a vibrational energy that was mild and pleasant. I suspect there was much more power underlying the effects than I was able to observe.

When it was my turn, Chief Joseph bowed his head respectfully as I chanted a traditional mantra of protection, together with the mantra blessing of abundance.

After the chanting, we sat together and spoke for a few minutes. Chief Joseph impressed me with his unassuming manner and his easy way of being with people, a quality I've observed in many teachers who understand the mystical forces that are always with us.

Christian Prayer.

There are many liturgical Christian prayers, such as the Kyrie Eleison ("Lord have mercy") and the Dona Nobis Pacem ("Give us peace"), which are part of the Roman Catholic Mass, the daily devotional services sung by monks, and Gregorian chants. Prayers like the Hail Mary, which are said repetitively, are also familiar to many Westerners.

Like mantra, Gregorian chant is a powerful method for awakening the mind and heart of singers and listeners to deeper levels of being. As scholar Katherine Le Mée writes in *Chant*, "Medieval people were well aware of the formative power of music. They knew that setting lines of scripture to song would imprint them ever more deeply into the memories of the worshipers, and that the words' effects would be sustained over longer periods of time, with greater intensity. They also knew that sound is causal, that it can bring about changes in the very nature and fabric of society as well as within the individual." Just as the repetition of mantras has the power to clear the mind and make it more responsive to the inner promptings of the spirit, so the repeated singing of Gregorian chants can ease the mind and be a salve to the spirit.

However, the significant difference between traditional Christian chants and mantras is that mantras are about energy. Mantras break up unhealthy or negative energy patterns stored in the physical and subtle bodies and help create new, positive energy patterns. This "clean" energy animates the body and mind and can act as a magnet for other positive energy to come into your life.

Kabbalistic Chanting.
The similarities between Jewish Kabbalistic thought and Vedic thought are quite remarkable. Just as the Sanskrit language is a key to spiritual knowledge and power, the same can be said for Hebrew. As H. P. Blavatsky writes in *The Secret Doctrine*, "In Sanskrit, as in Hebrew, every letter has its occult meaning and its rationale; every letter is a cause and an effect of a preceding cause. These linkages very often produce the most magical effect. The vowels, especially, contain the most occult and formidable potencies."

Abraham Abulafia, who lived in the late thirteenth century, was a heretic within Kabbalistic circles. He defied the secrecy that had been enforced for centuries by masters who sought to hide the power of the "names," or letters, in the Hebrew alphabet. Abulafia single-handedly made esoteric knowledge available to ordinary people for the first time.

Here there are some parallels with the Buddha, who swept aside secrets kept by orthodox Brahmin priests and made meditation practices, including mantras, available to all.

In his mystical book *The Pomegranate Orchard*, Moses Cordovero expresses the idea that manifestations of God's attributes descend into human consciousness in the form of sound. By linking themselves to these sacred vibrations, the prophets of ancient times came to see that all worlds, all stages of consciousness, and all beings are one.

This concept is almost identical to that handed down for thousands of years by the seers of India. However, there are great differences between the two systems in practice. For example, in the Vedic tradition the Sanskrit alphabet produces effects according to a very distinct biospiritual mechanism. Regardless of the desired result—whether attaining union with the Divine, asking that a loved one be healed, or finding a new job—the Vedic methods for chanting mantras are the same. En route to solving problems related to healing or resolving life issues, the sacred Sanskrit alphabet sounds produce a particular biospiritual effect. In the Kabbalistic tradition, the body is relatively insignificant. The chanting of mantras is often devotional and religious in nature, but there is also an ancient form of applied science behind the practices. These mantras are healing not only for the soul but for the body and mind as well.

Many traditions of chant from around the world are characterized by a deeply felt spirituality and a belief in the power of sacred sound to create change in everyday life. As you learn to use mantras in your own life, you may find your personal approach to using these ancient formulas takes on these characteristics. And you may also find that you want to keep your mantra private and personal, protected from the influence of others, just as many traditions have kept their chants and rituals secret.

2

How Mantras Work:
Our Spiritual Physiology

Over many years, I've found the centuries-old teachings about karma to be absolutely fundamental to my use of healing mantras. The Sanskrit word *karma* has entered the English language as part of our popular culture, but what does it really mean? Karma is the sum total of all our thoughts, actions, dreams, and desires that follow us from life to life through time and space, weaving the cords of our connection to the universe.

Why do things happen as they do? Why does one person succeed while another fails? Why does a particular individual recover from a seemingly terminal illness while another dies? Questions such as these have occupied philosophers and spiritual thinkers for thousands of years. Many different answers have been proposed, but more often than not no explanation has been fully satisfying to our spirits or our rational minds.

In the biblical story of Job, a bet between God and the devil inflicts terrible suffering on a thoroughly righteous man. But when the victim calls out for an explanation of what has happened to him, God replies that a mere human being has no right to ask. Nor does anyone have the capacity to understand the divine forces that govern the universe. God made the whale, he reminds Job, and until humans are able to perform a comparable wonder, they must accept their fate and not rail against it.

The classical traditions of Greece and Rome impart a similar message. In the *Iliad*, the epic poem of the ten years' war between Greece and Troy, a combination of immutable fate and frivolous domestic squabbles among the gods determines who dies and who survives. The gods often acted on their human subjects by assuming other identities and bodies, behaving, in other words, as karmic instruments of change, challenge, consciousness, and reward. While the Greeks and Romans could sometimes, through supplication, assuage the gods' mercurial emotions and actions, the gods' decisions were largely immutable.

The Vedic teachings about the practice of mantra, however, offer a direct way to affect the sea of circumstances in which we swim every day, throughout our physical lives. The masters believed that we humans can do something about our fate—with mantra.

Karma

Fate and karma are actually two very different ideas. Fate implies helplessness, the individual controlled by an immutable universe. Karma, on the other hand, is really an empowering concept. The Sanskrit word *karma* has entered the English language as part of pop culture. But what does it really mean? Very briefly, karma is simply the law of cause and effect. In the current vernacular it means "What goes around comes around"; in a biblical advisory, "As ye sow, so shall ye reap." What we send out into the universe will come back to us in some form—and this process can encompass even more than one lifetime.

Through the exercise of our free will, according to the Vedas, we both accumulate and "work off" karma, and the karma we draw to ourselves is both positive and negative. However, while "good karma" can be said to be preferred over "bad karma," the ultimate goal is to have no karma at all, at which point we are released from the wheel of rebirth and may transcend this earthly plane. Good karma, just like its opposite, actually attaches us to this plane.

Vedic teachings describe four types of karma:

1. **Sanchita karma** is the sum of all *accumulated past actions* in all of our *previous* individual lifetimes. This type of karma sets the stage for the present lifetime as well as, possibly, for others yet to follow.

2. **Prarabdha karma** is that portion of Sanchita karma that has resulted from *past actions* in this *present* lifetime. This type of karma concerns us most from day to day. While we cannot alter the events of this lifetime that have created Prarabdha karma, we can, with the practice of mantra, alter our inner conditions, both physically and emotionally, and thereby change the effect that Prarabdha karma has on us.

3. **Agami karma** results from actions in the *present* lifetime that will affect *future* incarnations. This type of karma can be thought of as sowing the seeds that will later be reaped. The Buddhist idea of "right livelihood," the Golden Rule, or the Ten Commandments, for example, can be used as guidelines in this lifetime for optimum karma in our next lifetime.

4. **Kriyamana karma** results *immediately* from our *present* actions. If, for example, you strike out at someone, he or she may very well strike you back. Kriyamana karma is "instant karma."

Storing Karma

Karma is carried with us like baggage that we store in various parts of the body. For example, Sanchita karma—all our past actions and decisions—is stored in the soul. At the moment of our birth, a portion of that total karma is released into the physical body and another portion goes into the subtle body. The rest of our total karma remains stored and will not come into play during this particular lifetime. The portions of Sanchita or past-life karma that have been released will be expressed through the network of neuron pathways that define the activity of our mind/brain and our personality, as well as our physical body. Sanchita karma will also affect our birth situation, presenting us with a predisposition and an environment that will influence our habits, prejudices, and the development of talents and abilities we will use in this lifetime to work off a given portion of our karma.

As we go through life, the people we encounter or circumstances we are met with will trigger individual bits of karma, releasing them and bringing them into play. When this happens we are presented with an opportunity to work off that particular portion of our karma. Let's say, for instance, that something bad happens—you are fired from a job, contract a serious illness, or lose a lover. One person may become depressed or discouraged, while another person, facing those same circumstances, may remain positive, or become even more determined to overcome the obstacle. Either person, however, will be working through his or her own particular karma.

Working with Karma

The word "mantra" derives from the Sanskrit words *manas*, or "mind," and *trai*, "to protect" or "to set free from." The literal meaning of mantra, therefore, is "to set free from the mind." Mantra is a mental tool that can release us from our conditioned mental habits and from the bondage of any predetermined life circumstances. The journey from mantra to freedom is rewarding and wondrous; it takes you beyond the static and stasis of everyday thought into the fundamental essence and oneness of consciousness.

The Law of Karma also includes the idea of grace, whereby negative karma may be forgiven by divine authority, or even taken on by someone else in order to serve some higher purpose. A most compelling example of this occurs in the New Testament, in which Jesus is said to have taken on the collective sins of humanity.

But the idea of taking on karma is by no means restricted to divine personages or religious figures. Highly evolved spiritual teachers have assumed the karmic burdens of others willingly. The great sage Paramahansa Yogananda once visited a place in India where elephantiasis was widespread. When he began to exhibit all the symptoms of the disease, Yogananda simply said that he was "doing his part," which his students understood to mean that he had taken upon himself a portion of the disease in order to ease the suffering of those who were afflicted.

I once complained to a spiritual teacher about a difficulty I was having. After looking me over he said, "Okay, let me have it." Something within me lifted, and he seemed to sag a little. "There's another agony put on me," he commented, wryly. But then he shrugged, as if to say, "Who cares, anyway? It's just the body and I am not this body."

Chanting mantras works directly on all types of karma, helping to overcome what may have been created inadvertently or ignorantly in this life or some past life. As part of the process, we can heal various physical, emotional, and spiritual conditions that we bring in to this life as part of our karmic inheritance. Chapter 6 provides numerous mantras for addressing planetary karma, including Sanchita and Prarabdha karma. If you are suffering the effects of Kriyamana and Agami karma at this time in your life, however, you may want to try the following mantra before you move on:

Om Sri Shanaishwaraya Swaha

(OM SHREE SHAHN-ESH-WAHR-EYE-YAH SWAH-HA)

"Om and salutations to Saturn, the planet of lessons."

In our everyday experience of the world, we take for granted the idea that we are separate individuals, distinct from our surroundings. When you look at a tree or a chair, you understand that those objects exist apart from you, the person observing them. The tree and the chair are in one place, and you are in another.

Similarly, if you look at a photograph of your parents that was taken before you were born, or if you read a book about the Civil War, you know that the moments they record took place in the past, and that the passage of time separates you from the realities these records depict.

In some important respects, however, this separateness is an illusion. If you stand in your backyard and stare at a tree, the tree exerts a gravitational force on your body that most definitely exists, although it's too weak for you to feel. The same gravitational force causes objects to fall to the ground rather than float off into space. The Moon exerts the same force on the Earth to create the tides. Through the force and energy of gravity, objects are actually in touch with one another despite their apparent physical separation.

Because of factors such as heredity and memory, we are not really separated from the past either. Things that happened long ago continue to affect us every day. At this very moment, our lives are partly determined by events that took place many years ago, before we were born. For instance, the light we see from stars winking at us from the blackness of the night sky emanated from those stars millions of years ago, and is only now reaching our planet. The very matter of which our bodies are made was formed at the dawn of creation.

In the previous chapter we examined the Pythagorean view that, by exposing ourselves to beauty and symmetry, we can assimilate the good energy of those qualities into our consciousness and even into our physical bodies. Just as a tree can be struck by a lightning bolt from the sky, the power of the cosmos can jump the gap between our individual, separate selves and the universe at large. One way to invoke this positive, beneficial energy flow is through the practice of mantra.

The Caduceus and Our Spiritual Physiology

Sound can alter our mood and improve our general well-being. Yet the key to understanding mantra lies in the relationship between our physical selves and our spiritual physiology, which many teachers of metaphysics refer to as the subtle body. The subtle body interpenetrates

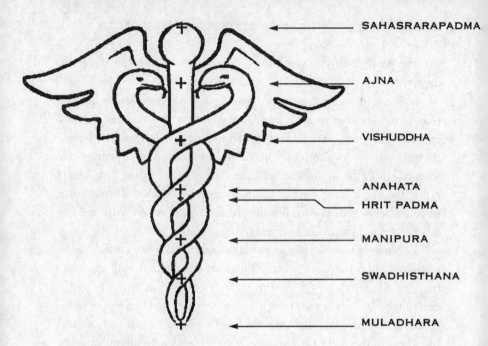

SAHASRARAPADMA

AJNA

VISHUDDHA

ANAHATA
HRIT PADMA

MANIPURA

SWADHISTHANA

MULADHARA

our physical body. It is an energy form that is an expression of both our individual body and the universal energy from which we and all material forms arose. The appearance and energy of the subtle body affects our physical and mental health and everything that we go through and experience. The subtle body influences the entire health of our physical body.

The ancient healing symbol called the caduceus beautifully illustrates the relationship between the physical body and the subtle body's spiritual physiology. A pair of serpents is twined around a central staff. At the top of the staff the serpents meet and wings sprout from their joining. In metaphysical circles, the caduceus is also known as the staff of Hermes, and it was once believed that its healing powers were capable of restoring vital energy to the dead.

Symbolically, the staff of the caduceus is the central axis of the subtle body and the spine of the physical body. The serpents represent the masculine and feminine currents—in Sanskrit, Ida and Pingala—that flow throughout the body, crisscrossing and meeting at five energy

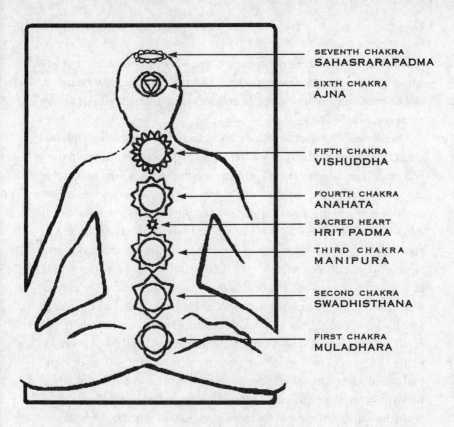

SEVENTH CHAKRA
SAHASRARAPADMA

SIXTH CHAKRA
AJNA

FIFTH CHAKRA
VISHUDDHA

FOURTH CHAKRA
ANAHATA

SACRED HEART
HRIT PADMA

THIRD CHAKRA
MANIPURA

SECOND CHAKRA
SWADHISTHANA

FIRST CHAKRA
MULADHARA

centers known as chakras, which are located physically along the spine. A sixth chakra is at the third eye, between the eyebrows, which connects us to a higher consciousness, in a union of human and divine intelligence. A seventh chakra exists at the top or crown of the head, where it mediates between the Divine and our higher consciousness.

Chakras

The Sanskrit word *chakra* means "wheel," and this is an apt image for the energy centers of our body. These energy centers resemble vortices, dynamic whirling forces in our subtle body. The chakras generally correspond with the major nerve ganglia or plexuses that act as localized miniature brains or "subprocessors" of information in our

physical body. Just as the nerve centers are working constantly to regu-
late our various physical systems, the chakras, too, are busy taking in
and distributing a basic energy, known as prana, throughout our physical and subtle body.

Some spiritual teachers have described the outer edges of the
chakras' energy whirls as resembling the petals of large vibrant sunflowers. Those adepts who are able to see the chakras, like those who
are able to see auras, also describe colors of various hue and intensity,
corresponding to the organs or parts of the physical body that each one
influences. The chakras' color, energy, and intensity vary according to
your state of health or disease. For instance, people who consume
large amounts of alcohol or drugs have certain characteristically unhealthy patterns. In such people, the chakra "flowers" may appear
almost lifeless, their colors muted. In fact, even in those of us in reasonably good health, the chakras normally resemble flowers drooping
on their stalks. In most of us, our chakras can hold and process only a
limited amount of energy. When we strive with mantra and other spiritual practices to strengthen our inner energy, and in particular when
we strive to awaken a dynamic form of energy called kundalini that lies
dormant within us, we can increase our chakras' capacity to hold energy, and optimize our health and well-being.

Although most books discussing chakras count six major chakras
located along the spine and one at the top of the head, there are really
dozens of chakras in the subtle body. Healers, for instance, often use
chakras located in the palms of the hands for the transmission of
pranic energy. There are chakras in the head that lie dormant and become active only when we grow to a certain stage of spiritual advancement. There are the two large chakras in the feet that can direct
energy outward in a powerful way when active in the advanced adept
or master.

Mantra works with the chakras in several ways. First, it clears
them of blockages so that they can function efficiently. Second,
mantras working in specific chakras "attract" energy from a usually
dormant feminine power cell in the first chakra located at the base of

the spine. This gives the chakras large amounts of energy to work with in restoring health, improving life conditions and circumstances, and eliminating karmic conditions that may have been hampering us in some way. Third, mantras draw on the ambient energy that is ever present around us but not available to the chakras. Through mantra formulas, we experience an actual net gain in our available, usable energy as well as tap the hugely powerful energy of kundalini. Chanting mantras is an especially effective way to activate energy throughout our body and spirit.

The five chakras located along the spine are:

1. **The Base Center: Muladhara chakra**
   PRINCIPLE: Earth
   Corresponds with the coccygeal plexus, the base of the spine or the anus, and governs the energy of elimination.
2. **The Sexual Center: Swadhisthana chakra**
   PRINCIPLE: Water
   Corresponds with the sacral plexus, the sexual and reproductive organs, which govern the energy of sexual activity, fertility, reproduction, and creativity.
3. **The Navel Center: Manipura chakra**
   PRINCIPLE: Fire
   Corresponds with the solar plexus, the stomach and abdominal organs, and rules the energy of digestive activities.
4. **The Heart Center: Anahata chakra**
   PRINCIPLE: Air
   Corresponds with the cardiac plexus, the heart, which governs the energy for circulation/respiration, and also supports the immune system.
5. **The Throat Center: Vishuddha chakra**
   PRINCIPLE: Ether
   Corresponds with the pharyngeal or laryngeal plexus, which influences the speech mechanism. This is also the "will" center.

6. The Brow Center: Ajna chakra
PRINCIPLE: Mind

Corresponds with the brain and its nerve centers, and is in the middle of the brow, between and slightly above the eyebrows. Also referred to as the third eye center. The sixth center is represented by the wings on the caduceus.

One last chakra that I wish to mention, but which is not on the spine or head, is known as the **Hrit Padma** or "sacred heart." It is located between the fourth and fifth chakras, three finger-widths below the heart in the front of the chest, and is considered in Vedic teachings to be the seat of the soul. In addition to the seven chakras and those in the hands and feet previously discussed, some spiritual leaders have taught there are also other, small chakras near the organs and glands.

Prana and Kundalini

In each of us, a primordial energy, prana, circulates, fueling all our various life-sustaining systems. There are really five kinds of prana: prana, upana, samana, udana, and vyana, but prana is generally known as the energy of spiritual light, which comprises the substance of our subtle body. Literally, *prana* means "breath." Without the flow of prana through our bodies, we would die. We direct prana with our minds when we do healing visualizations or mantra work. Pranic energy can be transferred from person to person, as healers do through their hands when they perform therapeutic massage, acupressure, therapeutic touch, reiki, jin shin jyutsu, and other hands-on treatments.

But kundalini energy is different from prana. Kundalini is an energy of spiritual evolution, growth, and consciousness, although it has been incorrectly viewed as a sexual energy. It can be compared to a dormant power cell located at the base of the spine at the first chakra. It has also been pictured as a snake coiled three and one-half times in quiet repose at the base of the spine. In most people, kundalini lies dormant as "energy in potential." We can, however, through spiritual practices such as mantra, prayer, and meditation, awaken this energy, causing it to move up the spinal canal, energizing the plexuses of the physical body and the corresponding chakras of the subtle body. According to mystical literature, the process begins gradually and proceeds through many years, or even lifetimes. Eventually kundalini energy will reach the brow center, or third eye. When that happens, cosmic consciousness or self-realization is achieved. In this new or additional state, healing abilities can manifest. Awareness increases so that the answers to deep spiritual mysteries are suddenly obvious. The interconnectedness of all life may become a visceral "knowing" instead of a mere concept, and we see the infinite results of our every action and thought.

Kundalini and higher consciousness can also become aroused spontaneously through events of everyday life. When you are deeply moved by a piece of music, or inspired by a poem, or when you feel deep love for another person, kundalini is beginning to awaken. Yet this partial manifestation is still only the "smoke." The "fire" of universal energy is quite different and indescribably intense.

While only a few of us may arrive at an exalted state of consciousness, we can all benefit from using mantras to energize our chakras and spirits.

Mantra practice helps to prepare the chakras to receive and use large amounts of spiritual energy. In most of us, the chakras can hold only a limited amount of spiritual charge. Filling them with a high charge coming from the kundalini without proper preparation would only be harmful. Therefore, kundalini experiences in which the energy is awakened by life experience or meditation are usually mild. There are, however, stories of people who have had fully charged awakenings that have changed their lives forever.

In the West, we have not been much exposed to this phenomenon, although the effects of such an awakening can be recognized in the healing works and life of Jesus. Christians speak of the power of the Holy Spirit to animate, heal, and enlighten. In our own times, those who have received a blessing from Paramahansa Muktananda can testify to the powerful current he transmitted to his initiates. Similar abilities were attributed to the nineteenth-century Hindu mystic Ramakrishna and his follower Vivekananda.

Mantra Increases Our
Spiritual Wattage

Mantra allows the chakras to "switch on" safely and to operate at a higher "wattage." When we practice Sanskrit mantra, we increase the ability of the chakras to hold a spiritual charge. It is as if a 25-watt bulb becomes able to hold 50 watts, then 100 watts, 500 watts, 1000 watts. Mantras' power derives not from any particular meaning that their syllables convey, but from the vibrational effect they create when they are pronounced repeatedly.

With this overall understanding of our spiritual physiology, of our subtle body and chakras, and of the way in which our deepest spiritual energies can awaken, we can now discuss what happens to us as we pronounce mantras. The process of intoning these ancient formulas works in the everyday world even if we don't understand what we are saying, because mantras are fundamentally about energy rather than meaning.

There are fifty letters in the basic Sanskrit alphabet. These letters correspond to the fifty petals on the six chakras from base to brow. Like the chakras themselves, advanced spiritual adepts can actually "see" the letters on the petals of the chakras. When a Sanskrit mantra is uttered, the petals corresponding to the letters contained in the mantra vibrate in spiritual resonance. This sets off a cascade of energetic effects.

First, the petal itself—the outer energy of the chakra—is stimulated by the vibration and becomes tuned to a higher energy state. Then, as a stone causes a ripple to travel across a pond, the petals of the chakra vibrate the energy of the corresponding plexus in the physical body. These vibrations have stimulating, strengthening, and regulating energetic effects that are healing to our physical systems. Just as lifting weights increases the ability of our muscles and even our skeletal structure to handle tasks requiring more strength, chanting Sanskrit mantras provides a workout for our chakras. We experience a net gain in our spiritual energy and a corresponding increase in our capacity to process powerful kundalini energy. Moreover, when we focus the sound vibration of mantra with a consciously held *intent*, we can even direct its energy (prana) to specific parts of the body.

Through the vibration of mantra, ambient spiritual energy is attracted to and gathered into the chakras of the chanter, increasing that person's total spiritual energy.

In addition to energizing the chakras and bringing in energy from the "near surround" (as they say in physics), mantra also balances the feminine and masculine energies that crisscross the body, allowing kundalini to flow through the body.

As the kundalini fills each chakra, the "sunflowers" begin to straighten on their stalks, their flowers no longer closed and drooping but fully opened and spinning with new levels of energy that provide even more vitality to the physical body.

What Goes Around Comes Around

As mantra stimulates and energizes the chakras, allowing them to take in and send out more energy to the subtle body and the physical body, there is yet another effect that is taking place: karma is being burned off. The vibration produced by chanting mantra begins to alter our inner condition, both physically and spiritually, and to break down energy patterns stored in the subtle body. These can be anything from subconscious habits or predispositions to a karmic potential for mishap. In most cases we are talking here about Prarabdha karma, karma we have accumulated through the past actions but are working within this lifetime. But it is also possible to burn off Sanchita karma (from past lifetimes) in this way.

Some Fundamental Truths to Remember about Mantra

1. **Mantras are energy-based sounds.** Words used in conversation derive their power from the meaning they convey. Mantra derives its power from the energy effect its sounds produce. Pronouncing a mantra creates a particular physical vibration in the form of sound that in turn produces various "energetic effects" in the physical and subtle body.

2. **Mantras are also chakra-based sounds.** Each of the fifty letters in the Sanskrit alphabet corresponds to one of the fifty petals on chakras one through six, from the base of the spine to the brow. Sanskrit mantra vibrates to the letters in the words of the mantra, which energizes the petal, and attracts ambient spiritual energy in the atmosphere to the person pronouncing the mantra. In this way, mantra affects both our physical bodies and our spiritual consciousness. We literally grow, in spirit and in flesh.

3. **Mantra—combined with intention—increases physical and spiritual benefits.** When we combine the physical energy of mantra, the *sound vibration*, with the mental energy of *intention and attention*, we increase, strengthen, and direct the energetic effect of mantra. Intention, the reason we are saying the mantra, is carried on the physical vibration, producing an effect. This is the essence of Sanskrit mantra.

4. **Mantras have only an approximate language-based translation.** If we warn a young child not to touch a hot stove, we try to explain that the stove will burn the child. However, language is insufficient to convey the experience. Only the act of touching the stove and being burned will adequately define the words "hot" and "burn" in the context of "stove." Essentially, there is no linguistic translation for the experience of being burned.

   It's the same with mantras. The only true definition is the experience that a mantra ultimately creates in the individual who chants it. Nevertheless, from the original "seer" of a given mantra to the shared identical experiences of those who have subsequently used it, a mantra will obtain an "experiential definition," that is, it will be known by the effect it produces.

5. **Mantra energizes prana.** Prana is our basic form of life energy that is capable of being transferred between individuals. Some healers operate through a conscious transfer of prana; a skilled massage therapist, for example, can often transfer prana with beneficial effect. Self-healing is also possible by concentrating prana in specific organs.

   When we pronounce a particular mantra while visualizing an internal organ bathed in light, the power of the mantra can become concentrated in that organ with great beneficial effect. The act of visualization, in this instance, works as intent, focusing and directing the energy produced by the mantra.

6. **Mantras are energy that can be likened to fire.** Fire can cook your lunch or it can burn down the forest. It's the same fire. Mantras, too, evoke powerful energies and should be treated with respect. There are even some powerful mantra formulas that must be learned and practiced under careful supervision by a qualified teacher. These are kept as closely guarded secrets and have not left the Far East.

   The mantras widely used in the West and those contained in this volume are perfectly safe to use on a daily basis, even with intensity.

Mantras and the Transformation of Consciousness

Human consciousness exists on many levels at once. It is really an intricate collection of states of consciousness distributed throughout the physical and subtle bodies. In fact, each organ of the body has a primitive consciousness of its own that allows it to perform specific functions. Each organ is also part of a system. The cardiovascular system, the reproductive system, the digestive system, and the nervous system all include organs working at slightly different stages of a single process. Similar levels of function and states of consciousness exist within the subtle body as well.

When we pronounce mantras, we initiate a powerful vibration that corresponds to both a specific spiritual energy level and a state of consciousness in seed form. Gradually, the vibration of the mantra begins to override all of the other lesser vibrations. These eventually become absorbed by the mantra. After a length of time that varies from person to person, the great wave of mantra stills all other vibrations within individual organs and systems. Ultimately, the individual will be in perfect harmony with the energy and spiritual state represented by and contained within the mantra.

The practice of Sanskrit mantra increases the vitality and energy-utilizing ability of the chakras in our subtle body and the organs of our physical body. As we grow proficient in mantra meditation, new experiences may begin to present themselves to us. Some people may begin to see auras—the bands of colored light that surround each of us like a halo. Others may find that a mysterious energy is now available through the hands or feet. You may find that your intuition becomes much sharper.

Just as there is a great variety of human abilities, so, too, there is great diversity in the application of this newly available energy. Many of us will heal physical problems, change undesirable life conditions, and eliminate negative karma.

Throughout our lives, the life energy of prana courses through our biospiritual system. The chakras whirl, collecting and distributing energy, and the physical organs perform their functions with the energy at their disposal.

Just as mantra cleanses and energizes the physical body, mantra repetition has a similar effect on the subtle body. Even speaking a mantra very softly influences the chakras that correspond to the nerve centers of the physical body. Just thinking a mantra—pronouncing it subvocally in your mind—can further the process of clearing away spiritual impurities, energizing the chakras, and burning off karma.

3

How to Use
Your Mantra

Spiritual disciplines are very precise in their structure and method. The mantra disciplines usually have a central purpose for their performance and a specific number of repetitions associated with accomplishment of the objective.

To achieve strictly spiritual objectives, the sheer number of repetitions can often seem impossible: 125,000 or more. But for solutions to worldly or material problems, the rules are quite different, and the repetitions far fewer. This chapter will help you put together a specific path for helping yourself and others through the mechanics of mantra practice.

Worldly Problem Solution

The best way to begin solving a problem is to state the problem clearly. Write it on a piece of paper. Even if you write just a few sentences, sketch the problem out as concisely as you can. Then fold up the paper and put it in a special place where it will remain as long as you are performing the disciplines: on top of a dresser, on a closet shelf, in a jewelry box, in a desk drawer, or elsewhere. If you decide to place your paper out in the open, then you might be moved to put some aesthetic objects nearby—candles, incense, pictures, crystals, or similar items. But you don't have to do any of this. Just your folded paper and a seriousness of intent will be quite enough.

Basic Approaches.

Now that you have prepared a simple foundation for your discipline, you can choose between one of two basic approaches:

- *Repetition of the mantra as often as possible over a specific amount of time.* This approach means that you will remember to say the mantra as many times as possible throughout each day. While doing household chores, you will say the mantra. In the shower, on a walk, while driving your car, you will say the mantra. Of course, be sure that you remain alert if you do mantra while driving. If you find that the practice of mantra while driving makes you "space out" then discontinue it at once.

  If you want to try this approach but are also curious about how many times you repeat a mantra during the course of a discipline, here is an easy way to keep track. Sit down with a watch, check the time, and repeat the mantra for five minutes exactly while counting how many you do. You can use your fingers or beads or whatever else you may prefer. Then multiply the result by twelve. You now have a figure for how many times you say the mantra in one hour.

  During the day, keep track of how many hours you say the mantra. It works like this: thirty minutes while driving my car, fifteen minutes while doing the dishes and clearing the sink, ten minutes while taking a shower or washing up, and so on. Keep a small notebook in which you record your daily amount of time in mantra repetition. At the end of the number of days you have allotted for the practice, add up the number of hours and multiply by the number of mantras you calculated as your rate per hour. You now have the number of mantra repetitions for the entire period. The minimum number of days for this kind of discipline is twenty-one.

- *Forty-day discipline.* A discipline of forty days is the time given for practicing mantra in the Eastern texts. As mentioned earlier, sages taught this process centuries even before Noah walked the earth.

Place.
In addition to saying your mantra as often as possible, you should set a specific place where you will practice your spiritual discipline twice every day.

Time of Day.
Set your practice at the same time every day. It is recommended that you perform your practice in the morning upon rising and in the evening before bed.

Traditionally, spiritual disciplines are performed at "the meeting of the day and the night," or *sandhya* in Sanskrit. This is a period lasting from two hours before dawn until dawn, and two hours before sunset until sunset. At this time, the Eastern scriptures teach, there is great spiritual energy streaming across the earth. While any time is appropriate for practicing mantras, the periods just before dawn and dusk are reported to be especially good.

Completing the Practice.
If you are in the midst of your discipline and the telephone rings, do not answer it. Better yet, before you begin, put on the answering machine or unplug the phone. You should strive to complete your daily disciplines without interruption.

Prayer Beads: Mala or Rosary.
If you wish, you can select a rosary or mala for your practice. If you decide to do so, put it in a safe place and use it only for this particular practice until you have completed the discipline. Alternatively, some people like to wear the rosary when they are not saying the mantra. This also is a good practice.

The rosary is an ancient spiritual tool. Throughout the Far East, rosaries are called malas and consist of 108 beads. For spiritual disciplines, rosaries are used the same way regardless of the religious tradition: primarily to count the number of repetitions of the mantra or prayer. While 108 beads had been used in Vedic malas for thousands of years before the birth of Jesus, the Catholic Church adopted fifty-four beads, one-half mala, plus a pendant consisting of five beads. (While this five-decade version is the most familiar, the "full" rosary consists of fifteen decades of beads plus the pendant.) One might say, for example, that one has performed twenty rosaries or ten malas of a specific prayer or mantra. As any practicing Roman Catholic can tell you, saying the rosary is a powerful experience.

One bead at the end of the mala is called the meru; it contains the accumulated power of all the mantra performed. (On the Catholic rosary, the pendant corresponds to the meru.) When using a rosary of either Western or Eastern variety, one should not "cross over" the end bead. It stores power. The Sanskrit word *meru* means "mountain." Spiritually, the meru becomes a "mountain" of stored spiritual energy. During your repetition of a mantra, the mala is finished when the meru is reached. To continue chanting the mantra, you start the count backward from the meru. Thus, in long sessions of mantra, the counting goes round the mala to the meru, then back again. Then forward round the mala again, and then back the other way to the beginning.

Most malas still contain 108 beads today. The number 108 is used because Vedic teachings state that there are 108 principal astral channels leading from the heart in the subtle body out to the rest of the subtle body. These channels can be likened to astral nerve tubes or blood veins. Saying a mantra 108 times sends energy into each of the channels.

There are malas made of several types of material in general use. These include:

- *Sandalwood.* Sandalwood is a general-purpose material that can be used for any spiritual discipline.
- *Tulasi* or *basil wood.* Basil is an herb widely used in Eastern and Western cooking. Some plants in the basil family can grow to be

quite large and their stalks quite wooden, making them a source
of wood for carved and sanded mala beads. Mantras invoking
the energies of Rama or Krishna, both manifestations of the god
Vishnu, are strengthened by using this material. Also, invoca-
tions of the feminine energies of Lakshmi and Saraswati are
aided with this material.

- *Plain wood.* In Tibet and other places where trees and thick veg-
  etation are the exception rather than the rule, malas are composed of the available material or imported. Thus, many malas
  made in Tibet and Nepal are of plain unnamed wood. They
  work very well for any purpose.

- *Rudraksha.* This is a small berry that hardens and can be drilled
  and strung. It is said to increase the power of mantras of Shiva
  (masculine) and Durga and Kali (feminine). It may also be used
  for Gayatri mantra, although *tulasi* and sandalwood are both
  more commonly used with the Gayatri, which is discussed in
  chapter 13.

- *Crystal beads.* Various types of crystal can be used to create
  beautiful malas, which also can become repositories of spiritual
  power. You can make your own malas or make them for others.
  They make wonderful gifts for the spiritually inclined.

Religious and Personal Images.

Some people like to put a picture or statue of a saint, or some other religious picture that is dear to them, next to their written mantra or the
place where they meditate. When doing healing work for someone
else, some practitioners like to place a picture of the person for whom
they are working in the meditation area.

Spiritual Diary.

I highly recommend keeping a spiritual diary. You may see or hear
things in your meditations to which you may want to refer later, even
years later. I have kept a spiritual diary at various times, and I wish I
had kept one all the time. We forget even things that seem indelible at

the moment. I have occasionally gone back over my dairies from years long past and seen and recalled things written there I had long since forgotten.

Any Mantra Will Do.
Strictly speaking, you can perform a spiritual discipline with any mantra. It can be one single mantra that you perform for one complete mala every day for forty days. This qualifies as spiritual discipline in the classical sense. But as with anything else in life, the more effort and concentration you apply, the more dramatic may be the results you derive. This is why nearly all disciplines are performed twice daily, once in the morning and once in the evening.

For those who have decided that they want a more intense discipline, the number of repetitions per sitting rises. Two malas twice per day. Five malas twice per day. Ten malas twice per day. Determine for yourself just how much time you will reasonably have each day, and give yourself some room.

Moving the Levers, Spinning the Dials.
Once you have started on a spiritual discipline, there will be consequences from your effort. Some of the consequences can be anticipated. Tensions may begin to ease. Or they may temporarily increase; this, too, is the result of clearing out negative energy.

It is not unusual for seemingly supernatural things to be heard or seen during the mantra practice. Please keep in mind that you have placed yourself in a situation where spiritual forces are at work. Sometimes the things experienced are relevant; sometimes they are random and irrelevant. The body is doing two things. First, it is bringing energy in from the spiritual "near surround" as well as processing kundalini energy through the chakras. Second, that new energy coming in is causing accumulated junk to be released and passed out from your energy world. As the junky energy patterns are releasing, they occasionally will cause thoughts or emotions to arise. As negative energy patterns pass from your body and your mind, you may experience them momentarily as they depart. Just know that anything that is truly important to you will be recalled when the meditation is complete. During your practice, honor what you see or hear but keep going.

You may see a flame, a patch of blue, or a five-pointed or six-pointed star. Usually you will become aware of these images at the center of your brow. Other mystical symbols may appear as well. I once saw a complex design very clearly. I did not know what it was until I saw the same design—the Sanskrit symbol for one of the chakras—on a book cover.

You may find there is a sudden obstacle to your practice. Probably at least once during your discipline, something will arise that will make it difficult to complete your discipline. Some event, problem, or circumstance will seem to be cause for you to miss a day or stop altogether. If at all possible, press on and complete the discipline. Try not to miss a day.

Many spiritual teachers from the East call these kinds of things tests. Perhaps they are, but I prefer to look at them as the result of a powerful force you have brought into play within yourself. There are parts of us that do not want to change—that actively resist change. These parts of ourselves can exert their influence in powerful ways, particularly when a countervailing force is applied to their habituated activity. The internal subconscious conflict created by a sincere and powerful spiritual discipline can be surprisingly sharp. If this seems foreign, then think of the person who has decided to quit smoking or to lose weight. Such people will tell you that they had to battle powerful inner forces that resisted any attempt at change.

When we practice mantra we are changing the nature of certain internal and usually crystallized energy clusters. They have become a part of our subconscious mind. They will invariably seek to assert themselves in some way to ensure their continued existence as they are. Continued practice of your mantra will mean that they must change in some way. Thus, some form of internal conflict arises.

Please know that these disciplines have been tested for thousands and thousands of years. If it is within your ability, press on with your discipline even if circumstances seem to militate against it. If it gets "too hot," then by all means stop, and try again at a later time. But it is best to keep doing your mantra. Do it every day without missing a day, if you can. Overall, things will improve, and sometimes quite dramatically, after you've completed the forty days. The specific condition that inspired you to undertake the discipline will be positively affected.

A Sample Spiritual Discipline

Here is an example of a sadhana, or strictly spiritual discipline, I once undertook.

The Maha-Mrityunjaya mantra is undertaken for longevity and for good health. A number of years ago, I became inspired to undertake this discipline in an entirely classical way, according to the Vedic traditions set down for it. This meant that I was required to repeat the mantra 125,000 times. I call this a freight train mantra because of its extreme length. Here it is:

Om Trayumbakam Yajamahe Sughandhim Pushti Vardanam Urvar-ukamiva Bandhanan Mrityor Muksheeya Mamritat

(OM TRY-UM-BAH-KUM YA-JAHM-MAH-HAY
SOO-GAHN-DIM POOSH-TEE VAHR-DAH-NAHM
OOR-VAHR-OO-KUMEE-VAH BAHN-DAHN-AHN
MRIT-YOUR MOOK-SHEE-YAH MAHM-REE-TAHT)

"Shelter me, O three-eyed Lord Shiva. Bless me with health and immortality and sever me from the clutches of death, even as a cucumber is cut from its creeper."

As a part of the discipline I was required to offer one-tenth of the total repetitions as water oblations for the sake of my ancestors. This will help mitigate any karma we have between us and also help them on their spiritual path. One-tenth of the repetitions must also be offered accompanied by spoons of clarified butter or oil in a fire ceremony, and one-tenth of the repetitions must be said while offering water oblations over my own head.

I completed the sadhana by working with it a little each week, but it took seven years. During the last portion of the sadhana, I found that I was able to write a book in just four months, and this led to a consulting assignment of great value. None of this was my objective. I was merely responding to an inner call to deepen my spiritual consciousness in a classical Vedic way.

I am certain that these unanticipated benefits came about due to the power of the mantra and my unwavering commitment to complete it, no matter how long it might take. You may very well find that completely unanticipated positive things come into your life, even if you are doing a discipline for someone else.

4

Seed Mantras

There are certain powerful, one-syllable mantras called seed mantras that have no explicit translation. In Sanskrit, these are known as *bija* mantras, and Vedic literature abounds with tales and legends of beings who used them and rose to greater heights of spiritual and material power. In the Rig Veda, for example, the earth spirit Kubera became the lord of wealth simply by chanting a few powerful seed mantras over a long (supernaturally long) period of time.

Unlike the words of everyday speech, bija mantras are experiences of energy in their own right. They are not symbols of other objects or experiences in the world. The word "chair" denotes an object with four legs, but seed mantras don't represent objects or even feelings. They're like the smell of a flower or the taste of an apple. Words don't define those experiences. The experiences define the words.

The Principal Seed (Bija) Mantras

If you have a particular issue in your life, or a material or spiritual goal you wish to accomplish, pick a seed sound that seems to represent the energy you desire but have been lacking. Work with this mantra for ten days, repeating it as much as you are able. Besides repeating it whenever you can, you should also consider setting aside five to ten minutes

twice a day to chant the mantra in a focused, meditative way. If it
agrees with you, continue for an additional thirty days. Then stop and
wait to see results (if they have not already presented themselves during your practice).

Shrim *[shreem]*.
This feminine seed sound is for the energy of abundance in all forms,
as expressed by the Sanskrit word *Lakshmi*, and personified as a goddess. Spiritual abundance, health, inner peace, financial wealth,
friendship, the love of children and family: Lakshmi is the source for
all of these, and the *Shrim* mantra is a powerful means of gaining any
of them. Repetition of the *Shrim* mantra gives you the ability to attract
and maintain abundance. According to Vedic teaching, if you pronounce *Shrim* a hundred times, your experience of abundance will increase a hundredfold. If you pronounce *Shrim* a thousand times or a
million times, the result is correspondingly greater.

Eim *[I'm]*.
This feminine seed sound rules artistic and scientific endeavors, music, and education. The name of this energy is Saraswati, a feminine
principle that at a deeper level governs the development and manifestation of spiritual knowledge. It is useful for achieving good education,
memory and intelligence, musical skill, and success in spiritual endeavors. Many Himalayan teachers have adopted Saraswati as part of
their spiritual name.

Klim *[kleem]*.
This seed mantra for the energy of attraction is neither masculine nor
feminine. It is often combined with other mantras to attract an object
of desire. To attract wealth, for instance, the abundance mantra can be
combined with the *Klim* seed to form the mantra *Om Shrim Klim
Maha Lakshmiyei Namaha*. Here *Klim* has been added to the regular
mantra *Om Shrim Maha Lakshmiyei Namaha*.
    Klim can also be used as a meditation. Find a quiet space where

you're unlikely to be disturbed, and begin your meditation by lighting a candle or a piece of incense. Sit comfortably and gently direct your thoughts toward the object or condition you desire to bring into your life. Or, visualize it as you would like it to occur or manifest in your life. As you do this, softly chant the mantra *Klim*. As you chant with this intention, you increase the energy of your thought and attract more energy to yourself.

Dum *[doom].*

This seed sound is for the energy of protection, which is also considered a feminine energy. If fear is a problem for you, this mantra will invoke protection and help you feel less afraid.

To begin, just chant the *Dum* mantra seed over and over whenever you feel in need of protection. You may chant it while you are going through your daily activities. If repetition of *Dum* becomes uncomfortable for any reason, stop for a while and then begin again later. After you are thoroughly comfortable with the *Dum* seed, lengthen the mantra to *Om Dum Durgayei Namaha*. This means "Om and salutations to she who is beautiful to the seeker of truth and terrible in appearance to those who would injure devotees of truth."

Krim *[kreem].*

This is the feminine seed of the Hindu goddess Kali, the goddess of creation and destruction. The powerful kundalini mantra *Om Krim Kalikayei Namaha*, which means "Om and salutations to the primordial feminine energy," produces an accumulation of power that can begin near the base of the spine or in the genital region. If you use this mantra and find that you have a shorter temper, then discontinue at once.

Also recall, from the discussion of *Klim*, that the mantra *Om Klim Kalikayei Namaha* can be used with good effect. Since *Klim* is the seed sound for attraction, it can also be used to attract Kali, or any other of the principles. In fact, some of the mantras presented later will include *Klim* as one of several bijas or seed mantras contained within the mantra.

Gum *[as in chewing gum]*.
This is a masculine seed for Ganapathi, an energy of the benevolent, elephant-headed god Ganesha, which removes obstacles and brings success in endeavors. To remove obstacles, repeat the seed mantra *Gum* for a few days until you are comfortable with it. Then move to the mantra, *Om Gum Ganapatayei Namaha,* which means "Om and salutations to the remover of obstacles for which Gum is the seed."

Glaum *[glah . . . owm]*.
Another seed for Ganapathi, this removes obstacles that may exist between the throat and the base of the spine. It is related to Ganesha as an energy of will.

Haum *[how, with an "m" added]*.
This is the seed for the abode of transcendental consciousness, a masculine energy manifested in the Hindu god Shiva, who is the personification of consciousness.

Kshraum *[an aspirated but unvocalized "k . . . sh," followed by a vocalized "rau," as in "how," and an "m" at the conclusion]*.
This masculine seed sound is for Narasimha, one of the manifestations of the god Vishnu. Narasimha has been used and invoked to be rid of the most stubborn evil situations. This sound releases your own pent-up energies. When you meditate on *Kshraum,* visualize the hidden power becoming available to you. *Kshraum* is also a seed for the destruction of seemingly indestructible demonic powers.

Hrim *[hreem]*.
This is a seed mantra for seeing through the illusion of everyday reality. According to various traditions, *Hrim* can be either masculine or feminine. You can find this seed mantra in both Vedic and Tibetan Buddhist practices, as part of longer mantras.

If a spiritual seeker practices this seed mantra devotedly and intensely just by itself, he or she will achieve clarity concerning the true reality of this universe. All illusions will be caused to fall away. The name of this feminine energy is Mahamaya, which is available through an energy center located just below the heart chakra. This energy resides within each of us, yet is not part of reality. The esotericists refer to it as the threefold flame. Followers of classical Vedic practices often call it the flame of Narayana, or "that from which this whole cosmos has sprung."

This flame can manifest material things as well as insights for you, here, on this plane of existence. Its fuel is devotion. It is also written in the ancient spiritual texts that this flame can put you in contact with higher realms where exalted beings dwell. If you are deeply devoted to a certain spiritual teacher who once lived, or to a particular tradition, this flame can actually manifest a likeness of that individual for you. You can use the seed sound *Hri* or *Hrim* as part of another mantra. If you meditate on the mantra *Hrim Shrim Klim Parameshwari Swaha*, the flame will eventually reveal a feminine form because "Parameshwari" is the Supreme Feminine. But if you envision, as the Tibetans teach, the syllable *Hri* within and meditate on the bodhisattva Manjushri, you will eventually see a male figure holding the sword of discriminating wisdom.

Chakra Bija Mantras

Gender-neutral bija mantras for the individual chakras help activate those chakras and prepare them for the handling of energy that is processed and used at that specific site. For instance, the seed sound *Ram* for the solar plexus chakra will produce smoother functioning of all the organs related to digestion.

Lam *[lahm]*.
Seed sound for the Muladhara chakra, located at the base of the spine. It is ruled by the Earth element and has the quality of smell. When a seeker meditates on *Lam*, a mystic fragrance is said to appear as an indication of spiritual progress.

Vam *[vahm]*.
Seed sound for the Swadhisthana chakra, located at the genital center.
It is a watery element and its quality is taste. While saying the *Vam*
bija, visualize a crescent moon over water. Patience will begin to manifest, as well as greater control of appetite and other senses.

Ram *[rahm]*.
Seed sound for the Manipura chakra, located at the solar plexus. The
ruling element is Fire and the quality is form. Meditate on *Ram* and
see a "friendly" fire that is part of you. When this energy becomes balanced, stomach ailments and digestive problems disappear.

Yam *[yahm]*.
Seed sound for the Anahata chakra, located at the heart center. The
ruling element is Air and the ruling quality is touch. Meditate on *Yam*,
the seed sound for the wind principle. You may hear music or the
voices of divine beings. (As the Bible says, if you encounter spirits, always test them.) Asthma and other lung disorders can be greatly re-
lieved by meditating upon this bija mantra.

Hum *[hoom]*.
Seed sound for the Vishuddha chakra, located at the throat center.
The element is Ether. The quality is sound. When you meditate on
Hum, illnesses of the throat are healed and languages become easy to
learn.

Om *[ohm]*.
Seed sound for the Ajna chakra, located at the third eye center. As described in chapter 2, masculine and feminine energies meet at the
third eye center. Thus, this seed sound contains the Principle of Unity.
There is a quality of cosmic intelligence associated with this seed
mantra. Through meditation on *Om*, worry is extinguished and the
mind becomes serene.

Each seed mantra has a unique power that you must experience individually. The ways in which they can work and manifest for you will differ greatly from the ways they work for other practitioners; this is to be expected given our many profound karmic and personal differences. Be open to whatever images or results the mantra delivers to you. Whatever changes occur in your life may contain the seed to the solution or goal for which you have been practicing mantra.

5

Mantras and Attracting Love

The Nobel Prize–winning physicist Richard P. Feynman once made an observation that he believed was applicable to material reality on every scale. Feynman said that all matter is naturally attracted to other matter, but only up to a point. When two objects get close enough, the energy of attraction for some reason transforms itself into resistance against further approach. The magnetic pull turns into a push. The force of gravity turns into antigravity.

How mysterious, but how true! You don't have to be a quantum physicist like Feynman to recognize this paradox, because you've probably seen it at work in your own relationships with other people. Though we long for intimacy, we want autonomy as well. Once we achieve real closeness, a desire for distance often asserts itself, causing us to damage or even destroy our relationships.

Plato, in his dialogue on love known as the *Symposium*, uses the metaphor of an egg to describe the seemingly impossible contradictions that are built into human relationships. Perhaps the two sexes were originally one harmonious entity, a character in the *Symposium* theorizes, just as an egg is a single, elegantly formed object. But once the egg has been broken, it cannot be put back together again. Still, we yearn to reunite the male and female energies in one entity; each woman or man longs for the other and hopes for an enduring relationship with another person.

I'm much more optimistic than either Feynman or Plato. I would hold that there is hope for any one of us seeking a lasting love. And mantra can be a powerful tool to achieve this. But, as with all other applications of mantra, achieving the desired result is dependent upon the quality of intention, and when it comes to finding a satisfying relationship with another person, it is of the greatest importance to begin with a clear understanding of what your goal should be.

The Ideal Other

When we set out to find a partner each of us is operating with a given set of criteria, a kind of blueprint or list of the characteristics that we want in a mate. Here in our Western world, for example, women in general would probably list that they want a man to be a good provider, a good companion, and perhaps a protector for them and their children. Women also want a man who can "turn them on" (though this criterion can certainly be met by a wide range of attributes). If a woman considers her spirituality to be an important aspect of her life, she may add that she is looking for a man who shares her spiritual sensibilities.

Men, I would have to say, would probably have at the top of their list that they want a woman who is physically attractive. Then they'd want someone they could "spend time with," although, frankly, I think many men have only a vague idea about what that would actually mean day to day. Many corporate businessmen still look for a supportive woman who can help them climb the ladder, and may limit their vision to someone who is good at entertaining and is of course "presentable," although some men don't mind if their wives have competitive, dynamic careers. Last, they might hope for a mate who is a "good mother." A man with spiritual leanings might add to his list of important items "conduct," "ethical values," and "morality."

But are these qualities reliable indicators of a good partner? Compared to the Vedic teachings, much of the Western notion of relationship is based on superficial qualities. The sacred writings of India provide us with a very different way of valuing one another, one that is more likely to bring lasting happiness.

Power Is a Feminine Principle

In the sacred writings of India, consciousness is described as a masculine attribute, and power a feminine. Until the feminine and masculine aspects come together, the universe exists only as potential. It is from the dance of Shiva, the masculine energy, powered by the feminine energy of Shakti that the universe is created.

Fire, with its power to burn, is often used in the East as a metaphor for the duality of the masculine and the feminine. The idea of fire is said to be masculine, but the power to make real flames is feminine. Without the feminine power, fire is merely an abstract idea without tangible existence.

The idea of power as a feminine attribute is unusual to us in the West, where for the most part our images of power are male-oriented. Yet the Eastern texts quite clearly describe Shakti as dynamic female energy and Shiva as a sleeping, or dormant, masculine consciousness that must be awakened. The creation of all matter and being occurs because the male energy has been ignited by the female. As a Vedic text declares, "Only when Shiva is united with Shakti does he have the power to create." Only with feminine power can the masculine idea of "fire" produce heat and light.

Mantra can help awaken and bring into balance these masculine and feminine energies and help the seeker attract an appropriate partner. It enhances the positive qualities of both male and female energies, and it refocuses them if they have been misdirected. When used by one or the other partner in a relationship, mantra heals and nurtures the spirits of both partners. When used to find or begin a relationship, it strengthens the attractive power of an individual, just as an electric charge can turn an ordinary piece of metal into a magnet.

In the West, the most famous Hindu treatise on sex is the Kama Sutra. *Kama* is Sanskrit for "desire." The Kama Sutra is only part of a body of knowledge and wisdom about sex, sacred sexuality, and the joyful spirituality invested in human form and function. Another part of Hindu teaching about sexuality is called Tantra. Female sexual energy in particular was described in Tantric teachings as the source of both sexes' attraction. As "one candle can light another," the awakened energy of the woman was invoked to awaken and arouse the energy of a man.

It was an axiom of Tantric belief that female energy cannot be stolen or extracted against a woman's will. This is a controversial statement, since men have a long record of exerting their force over women. But it is true that a woman's power is a blessing that she confers on a man if and when she chooses.

A scripture known as the *Kularnava Tantra* tells of the need for a quality of consciousness and intention to be brought to the practice of sexuality.

If merely by drinking wine men were to attain fulfillment, all addicted to liquor would reach perfection.

If mere partaking of flesh were to lead to the high state, all the carnivores in the world would deserve intense merit.

If liberation were to be insured by sexual intercourse with a shakti, all creatures would become liberated by female companionship.

—Kularnava Tantra
(translated by Mike Magee)

The power of the feminine is evident throughout the natural world.

I once saw a documentary film that provided a dramatic example of feminine power in action. A male lion was climbing toward a den of cubs sired by another male. He intended to kill the cubs, as male lions sometimes do to promote their own genetic line. Suddenly, the cubs' mother emerged from the den, stopping the male in his tracks. He hesitated, and lifted one paw, as if considering what to do. Meanwhile, the lioness lowered her head until her spine was absolutely straight. She looked the intruder in the eyes and bared her fangs.

The male lion clearly outweighed her by eighty to a hundred

pounds; ordinarily a fight would have been no contest. But when the lioness lowered her head, a straight channel of pure energy was created from the base of her spine to her eyes. The male took one look into those eyes, then turned and bounded away. Her energy had simply overpowered him.

As a resource for protecting her young, nature has given the female of every species ready access to a power that is much less accessible to males. In women, this energy is awake and functioning. In most men, it is not.

But what does that mean to the Westerner, for whom strength and action are identified with men? What should women look for in a mate if they are to be truly happy? What should men value in a partner? How can we find a truly spiritual partner? In this chapter, we will refer to power as a feminine principle, and we will explore how people of both sexes can help themselves find partners who are right for them.

The Predicament of the Sexes

In the West, the idea of a powerful woman is often tinged with resentment and fear. The Bible is one of the most important sources for our patriarchal tradition, and it abounds with portraits of women—from Eve, presumed to have caused humanity's exile from Paradise, to Delilah, betrayer of Samson—who are presented as undeniably strong but threatening and destructive. Greek and Roman mythologies also present an array of troublemaking women, both human and divine. The Trojan War's beginnings are attributed to the jealous rage of the goddesses Athena and Hera against Aphrodite, goddess of beauty.

Westerners' representations of women have, in my opinion, eroded solid, mutually respectful, working relationships. While both the Bible and the classical mythologies present many positive and heroic female characters as well, these women are not seen to empower men as those in the Vedic tradition do. In the Vedas, true feminine power is not the ability to manipulate or seduce. Feminine power is giving rather than taking. It imparts energy rather than steals it. A strong

woman wants to find a sharing, committed relationship, with a partner who can receive her energy in a positive way. But finding such a
partner can be difficult. And men, too, have trouble finding the right
partner.

Therefore it should not be surprising that one of the questions I
am asked most often is how to find the right or most compatible or
perfect mate or partner. I am also frequently asked how to find a spiritually compatible mate by individuals looking to integrate their spiritual practice into all aspects of their lives. After working for more than
twenty-five years with men and women who are looking for partners, in particular looking for spiritual partners, I have observed that
there are more available women who are spiritually oriented than
men. Nevertheless, mantra can help any woman or man find lasting love.

When a Woman Seeks a Man

From a Vedic perspective, contemporary women must ask, "Where
can I find a man who will honor me and respect my power, who will
use my energy honestly and unselfishly, without anger or resentment?"

I offer here a reliable mantra for empowering a woman to find
such a man:

Sat Patim Dehi Parameshwara

(SAHT PAH-TEEM DAY-HEE PAH-RAHM-ESH-WAH-RAH)

*"Please give to me a man of truth who embodies
the perfect masculine attributes."*

Intention:
Know What You Truly Want

I once knew a woman named Carol who was unhappy about the lack of a fulfilling relationship in her life. When we discussed what kind of man Carol was seeking, she used the same word over and over again. She wanted to find a "spiritual" man. Although she found it difficult to elaborate on exactly what this word meant to her, it seemed to me at the time a worthwhile, sincere aspiration.

I taught her *Sat Patim Dehi Parameshwara*, and she chanted this mantra for two weeks.

At the end of that time, she reported to me that she had met three men.

It sounded like real progress. "Great," I said.

"Not really," Carol said. "Every one of them was a bozo."

Bozo? It seemed an unlikely characterization for a spiritually oriented person to apply to another human being, but I didn't address it. Instead I pointed out that two weeks was probably not enough time to achieve the result she was looking for. Oddly enough, at almost the same time I was introduced to another young woman, Didi, who was having the same problem. She, too, wanted a "spiritually evolved" partner. But when I taught her the mantra, she soon returned with similar disappointing news. She had met two men. One of them, she also said, strangely enough, was a bozo, and one of them was "nice enough" but not really her type.

I suggested to both Carol and Didi that they continue to use the mantra in a very disciplined fashion for the traditional period of forty days. Neither of them was prepared to do this, however, and this puzzled me. Wasn't the creation of a fulfilling relationship important enough to concentrate on the mantra for a month or so? Finally I concluded that neither of them, deep down, really wanted to meet anyone—and five years later, neither of them had.

I also realized that there was a lesson for me in this experience: I should have realized that Carol's and Didi's vague descriptions of what kind of man they wanted to meet indicated they really didn't know what they were looking for. Since they themselves weren't clear in their intentions, the mantra could only attract unsatisfactory options for them.

I was reminded of a quote from Abraham Joshua Heschel: "When I was young, I admired clever people. Now that I am old, I admire kind people." And just as suddenly, Jimmy Stewart as Elwood P. Dowd in *Harvey* echoed in my head, "There are two ways of getting along in life: to be smart, or to be pleasant. I prefer to be pleasant." Now, I think it's perfectly possible to be both, but if I had to choose one, I'd choose pleasant.

But what would Carol choose? Or Didi? Would they value "smart" over "kind"? Would they expect spirituality to be handsomely packaged? Did they really want to accommodate themselves and their schedules to the daily give-and-take and compromise of a relationship? The mantra had answered their stated desire by attracting the energy of several men, but either their expectations or their indecision may have prevented them from seeing the possibilities for a real relationship.

Another woman with whom I worked, Linda, didn't need me to define what she wanted, which she said was a relationship based upon mutual respect and affection. In her early fifties, she had not been in a mutually committed relationship for more than five years, although she thought she was now ready to have one. But she did not know how to put forces into motion to bring that about. She had no interest in singles bars, or in trying to meet Mr. Right at the gym.

At my suggestion, we spent about ten minutes together in meditation, during which I chanted several mantras including the one given above. I taught her the mantra and asked her to continue to meditate on this goal as she practiced the mantra herself. Thirty days later, when I saw her again, she was positively beaming. She had begun seeing someone and was in the happy, early stages of a promising new relationship. As of this writing, Linda has been seeing this man for eight months and all is well.

What's the Rush?

Although it is possible to meet a man or a woman with whom we feel an instant intimacy, this is fairly rare, particularly if we are looking for someone with spiritual qualities, which are often inward, quiet characteristics. The fact is, true intimacy takes time to establish. This is why a period of getting to really know the other person—a period of courtship—is so important. Through mutual exploration in a variety of circumstances, both parties have the opportunity to discover the genuine qualities of the other.

The *I Ching* (the Chinese oracle-in-a-book) says that the path to happiness and spiritual advancement begins with uncompromising truthfulness with oneself in all matters. Truthfulness is the basis of real intimacy. When we experience intimacy, we are really experiencing the closeness that honesty brings. In any relationship, each of us must decide how intimate we want to be. Are we able to handle the intensity of truth with a partner? Will we be unsatisfied without it?

Here is a mantra that I use when I want to clear my mind so that I can consider these questions—or questions of any kind—in a placid and unobstructed state.

═══════════════════════════════════

Hung Vajra Peh

(HOONG VAHJ-RAH PAY)

*"By the power of will, through the spoken word,
I invoke the thunderbolt of my mind."*

═══════════════════════════════════

This Tibetan mantra is capable of clearing any space of negativity, whether physical, mental, or emotional. It is very helpful in giving you room to consider difficult questions of intimacy and true intention.

When a Man Seeks a Woman

Men often have the same kind of problem finding the right relationship. A young man named Howard was still hurting from a relationship
that had been completely over for several months. When I met him, he
was working as a security guard at a local bank. Howard had studied
martial arts and had evolved a general, spiritual practice and perspective that was very close to my own. I felt a kindred spirit. The bank job
was a way to pass the time while he recovered from losing the woman
he had greatly loved and while he decided what he wanted to do with
the rest of his life. He was also trying to decide what kind of relationship he wanted. I mentioned my work with mantra, and he soon asked
if there was a mantra that would help him.

Since Howard was hurting from the loss of feminine energy in his
life, I offered him this short, powerful mantra that expresses the feminine or Shakti energy of the universe:

Om Shrim Shriyei Namaha

(OM SHREEM SHREE-YEI NAHM-AH-HA)

*"Om and salutations to the creative abundance
that is the very form of this universe."*

Howard learned the mantra on the spot, right in front of the bank,
and started chanting it immediately. When I stopped by the bank later
that week he told me that he had chanted for half an hour the first day,
two hours the next day, and, that day, he had been chanting it all day
long. He said that it made him feel a bit odd, but he liked it.

Another week passed before I returned to the bank, at which time
Howard described an interesting incident. He had been talking on the
telephone with a woman who was an acquaintance but not a friend.

He was about to say good-bye, but to his surprise she asked if they could talk a bit longer. The woman sensed Howard's surprise but said that he seemed different somehow, and she was enjoying speaking with him.

Howard was certain that this was a result of the mantra, and I agreed. Howard was confident that the mantra would help him open to new opportunities in his life. He had already increased his own inner feminine energy, which created a powerful affinity with women who would previously have felt no energy at all coming from him.

The mantra I taught Howard will almost always result in a man's attracting a woman who will be compatible with him.

Another powerful mantra is also very effective for helping a man to find a woman:

Narayani Patim Dehi Shrim Klim Parameshwari

(NAH-RAH-YAH-NEE PAH-TEEM DAY-HEE SHREEM
KLEEM PAH-RAHM-ESH-WAH-REE)

"Oh power of truth, please let me attract a spouse carrying the supreme feminine energy manifesting abundance and creativity."

This mantra, employing the seed sounds for attraction and abundance, entreats the power of the flame at the Hrit Padma (Narayana) to provide a woman who holds the highest of the various feminine attributes, including abundance.

Mantras for Healing a Relationship

Healing a relationship by means of a mantra begins with both parties deciding to treat each other with mutual respect and committing to each other that they will work together to resolve their differences. The odds for success drop considerably if only one party in the relationship is engaged in the effort. If you work earnestly on the relationship but your mate takes a wait-and-see attitude, it's unlikely that you can work things out. In such a case, it is likely that the wait-and-see person is destined to move on in the near future—or he or she may simply continue whatever behavior is contributing to the problem.

In the beginning, you should sit down together and pledge to each other that you want to try honestly to better your dealings with each other. Then, you should conduct your mantra meditation separately for about ten minutes a day. Generally, each of you will experience insights and mini breakthroughs as you practice the discipline. Meditating separately facilitates the emergence of these insights. Set aside enough time each day to complete each mantra 108 times for forty days. The practice usually takes about ten minutes per day. At a minimum, you will need to practice for three weeks.

Two mantras are given here, one for honoring the feminine energy within each partner and one for honoring the masculine energy within each partner. The practice of mantra helps balance these inner energies of the individuals, enabling them to become harmonious as a couple.

To honor your feminine energy:

Hrim Shrim Klim Parameshwari Swaha

(HREEM SHREEM KLEEM PAH-RAHM-ESH-WAH-REE SWAH-HA)

"Salutations to the Supreme Feminine. May that abundant principle which hides the nature of ultimate reality be attracted to me."

This mantra contains great feminine power in a very simple form. By saying it as part of a commitment to a relationship, either party will purify his or her feminine energy and begin to accumulate usable, clean energy. It is significant that in certain branches of Shaivism, a Hindu sect honoring the masculine consciousness, this feminine-oriented mantra is chanted as the principal spiritual discipline. Some of these mantras were presented in chapter 4, but it's worthwhile to look at them again here:

Hrim is a seed mantra for dissolving the illusions of our perceived reality. It enables us to behold the world "as it really is." *Shrim* is the seed mantra for the principle of abundance in all forms. Now we are asking for an abundance of positive energy in the relationship, expressed in thoughts, feelings, and actions. *Klim* is the seed mantra for attraction. Here we intend it to attract whatever is needed to heal the relationship. *Parameshwari,* the Supreme Feminine, is invoked when we seek the abundant feminine spiritual energy of the universe to bless our efforts with success. *Swaha* means "I offer," or "salutations." By recognizing the great power of feminine energy and humbly offering gratitude, we sanctify the use of this power for our good intentions and purposes.

To Honor the
Masculine Principle

The Siddha mantra below will help both parties purify their masculine aspect. It is said that if one uses this as a main spiritual discipline for many years, one will eventually accumulate knowledge and spiritual clarity of the deepest type.

Om Nama Shivaya

(OM NAH-MAH SHEE-VAH-YAH)

*"Om and salutations. May the elements of this
creation abide in me in full manifestation."*

Healing Misunderstandings
in a Relationship

Misunderstandings can occur fairly often even in good relationships.
To resolve misunderstandings, you can use mantras to help you gain
your own clarity of mind in the midst of emotional and mental turmoil.
Two mantras invoking the Hindu divinities Subramanya and Ganesha
are particularly good for accomplishing this.

Focusing the Mind.
Subramanya is often referred to as the god of war in the Vedic pantheon. Historically, the concept of Subramanya derives from the razor-
sharp state of mind required for success in combat. But Subramanya
also has a wider application. To deliver us from confusion, the mind
must be strong, focused, and surrounded by good intentions. The following mantra, considered a good-luck charm by some of its ardent
users, invokes Subramanya under an alternate name. By repeating the
mantra you begin to focus your subconscious along optimistic lines,
and to clear out emotional debris so that you can function more effectively. As extraneous concerns are cleared away, you can see to the
heart of your misunderstanding. You can once again recognize your
partner's good qualities as well as your own strengths. With goodwill
and a clear desire for a relationship that works, you can gain the
courage to resolve your disagreement.

Om Sharavana Bhavaya Namaha

(OM SHAH-RAH-VAH-NAH BHAH-VAH-YAH NAHM-AH-HA)

The term *Sharavana Bhavaya* can literally mean "One born in the arrow-shaped forest grass" as Subramanya was. But the real meaning of the mantra is *"Salutations to the son of Shiva, who brings auspiciousness and who is chief of the celestial army."*

Resolving Inner Conflict.
Among the Vedic gods and goddesses, the elephant-headed divinity Ganesha is renowned as a remover of obstacles. Ganesha's mantra, below, can help you resolve inner conflicts that you may be projecting onto external situations. By helping you discern a state of mind that is creating disharmony between you and your partner (or between you and a friend or colleague), Ganesha produces order in the outer world. The tangible effects often seem like a sudden, almost magical disappearance of obstacles.

Ganesha is also known as Ganapathi. *Gana* means "power" in Sanskrit, and *pathi* means "spouse." So, in one context, the literal translation of the name is "spouse of power."

Gana can also mean "group" if used in another context. *Ganapathi,* then, becomes "spouse of the group." The power of this mantra will always be operational whenever people come together as a group. There is a correlation here to the words of Christ, when he said, "Wherever two or three are gathered in my name, I will be in their midst." Here is the mantra:

Om Gum Ganapatayei Namaha

(OM GUM GUH-NUH-PUH-TUH-YEI NAHM-AH-HA)

*"Om and salutations to the remover of
obstacles for which Gum is the seed."*

You and your partner can use either or both of these mantras to achieve mental clarity, to avoid and overcome misunderstandings, and to get your relationship back on track.

*Spiritualizing
Your Relationship*

Bringing a sense of spirituality into your relationship can be easy if you both love and respect each other and want the relationship to continue to grow. These qualities and intentions are prerequisite for a spiritually fulfilling relationship.

To enhance your feelings of intimacy and connection, you and your partner should meditate together for ten to fifteen minutes a day. It is an old maxim that when people meditate together, whether it is two people or two hundred people, their energies will automatically begin to harmonize and increase. After only two or three weeks of activity, the results should begin to show. You may feel a growing sense of peace between you, or a dynamic energy. Sometimes you may become so attuned to each other that you pick up each other's thoughts in the meditation. During the day, you may begin to finish sentences for each other in a loving way, and sense your partner's thought patterns and moods.

If either of you is holding any hidden or underlying hostility toward the other, joint meditation will quickly bring this to the surface. You should address any hurt, resentment, grievance, or other negative junk openly, caringly, and seriously. You need to try and heal this old business. Sometimes professional counseling or therapy may be needed. I have seen cases, over the years, where a couple began to meditate together and within thirty days discovered several issues to which they needed to give attention. This is a good thing. All of us need counseling from time to time, even if it's just talking about things with a friend.

Masculine and Feminine Invocations

According to Vedic tradition, a duality of masculine and feminine energies pervades all creation, from the distant galaxies to subatomic particles. Regardless of your sex, these same male and female forces are present in you as a human being. To fully realize yourself as a complete person, you must recognize these dual energies, honor them, and develop them within. Therein lies both your fulfillment and your freedom.

To enhance your feminine energy and its attendant power, purity, and authority as creative force, giver of birth, and protector of the young, choose one of the following mantras to chant.

Hrim Shrim Klim Parameshwari Swaha

(HREEM SHREEM KLEEM PAH-RAHM-ESH-WAH-REE SWAH-HA)

"Salutations to the Supreme Feminine.
May that abundant principle which hides the nature
of ultimate reality be attracted to me."

Om Dum Durgayei Namaha

(OM DOOM DOOR-JAH-YEI NAHM-AH-HA)

*"Om and salutations to she who is beautiful to the
seeker of truth and terrible in appearance to those
who would injure devotees of truth."*

Om Tare Tuttare Ture Swaha

(OM TAH-REH TOO-TAH-REH TOO-REH SWAH-HA)

*"Om and salutations. May the Mother of All
guard and protect me and fulfill my needs."*

Om Mata, Om Mata———,
Mata Jagadamba

(OM MAH-TAH, OM MAH-TAH———,
MAH-TAH JAH-GAH-DAHM-BAH)

*"Om Mother, Om Mother. Salutations to [insert your
favorite feminine principle, e.g., Mother Mary, Isis,
Aphrodite, Saraswati] who is a mother to the world."*

To enhance your masculine energy and its focused consciousness,
choose one of the following mantras to chant.

Om Nama Shivaya

(OM NAH-MAH SHEE-VAH-YAH)

*"Om and salutations. May the elements of this
creation abide in me in full manifestation."*

Om Namo Bhagavate Vasudevaya

(OM NAH-MOH BHAHG-AH-VAH-TEH VAH-SOO-DEA-VAH-YAH)

*"Om is the name of the Indweller in me that is ever in unity
with all of creation. Kindly reveal your truth to me."*

Om Ram Ramaya Swaha

(OM RAHM RAH-MAH-YAH SWAH-HA)

*"Om and salutations to that perfection in the physical realm which
was Rama, whose attributes exist in me also. Kindly manifest."*

If none of the above seems quite right, then turn to chapter 13, on the Gayatri mantra, the universal nonsectarian mantra on spiritual light, and follow the guidelines for practicing this great mantra.

My wife, Margalo, and I know that we are together not only to grow spiritually, by learning from one another as we go through life, but also for a higher purpose, which we interpret as being of service to all of humanity through our work and relationships with others. No matter what obstacle or misunderstanding occasionally intrudes itself into our life, we view it as a cloud passing in front of the sun. We know that it is merely illusory. We accept each other's great qualities and some flaws, knowing that while we still occupy this body we will face challenges in dealing with each other. Yet we face these challenges together, *with* each other, partly because of our mutual commitment *to* each other and partly because we know how to turn to mantras for help.

For my part, whenever we have a dispute or disagreement, I make time to meditate on the issue as soon as possible. My objective is to identify the improper mental or emotional condition I have brought to the dispute. Invariably my meditations reveal some long-standing unhealthy response pattern or false assumption. If the internal condition I have found is serious, I undertake a mantra discipline lasting from ten to forty days, with the intention of transforming that condition. Over the years I have achieved very good results with this practice. One outcome I have observed is that as I discard distortions within, Margalo's manifested shakti, a part of which is with me at all times, changes positively to help empower this new energy state.

For her part, Margalo works nearly every day with the twelve mantras of the sun and with scientific breathing practices (pranayama) to solve issues that she determines need work.

We come together to perform the ancient Sanskrit water and fire ceremonies that clear up any remaining energy debris. This practice has been very effective for us for many years.

6

Mantras for Changing
Physical and Planetary Karma

Many public figures, including U.S. presidents and their wives, have from time to time received advice from astrologers. Nancy Reagan sought to ensure that major policy decisions were made at favorable astrological times. Jefferson and Madison routinely checked the position of the planets for themselves and for the nation. Similarly, and often unbeknownst to their stockholders, many major corporations have astrologers on their payrolls, usually listed blandly as "investment consultants." Astrologers in towns and cities of every size analyze the position of the planets for their favorable, challenging, or downright difficult effects upon every imaginable kind of endeavor and enterprise.

In India, astrology has been integral to decision making since ancient times. Marriage dates are fixed according to planetary alignments that are favorable to the union of the two souls. Business deals have their mundane charts cast to ensure that the deal won't become difficult or even disastrous. A potential purchase date for a new home is scrupulously examined from an astrological standpoint. The best planetary alignments and correlations are arduously sought out and then acted upon.

Yet only Sanskrit mantra offers you techniques for counteracting the tendencies indicated by your natal chart. The Brahmin holy men of old would chant long sets of mantras for each of the planets and perform complex Sanskrit ceremonies designed to offset difficult alignments found in the birth charts of templegoers. Of course, priests were paid to do these ceremonies, so those who could not afford to pay got no help. But now the power of mantra is no longer controlled and regulated by a priestly class.

In this chapter you will find ways to mitigate many difficult alignments that astrologers may have told you exist in your natal or progressed chart. By chanting these mantras, you have the ability to change your karma, particularly karma that manifests in your body as illness.

Review: Types of Karma

As we discussed in chapter 2, there are four types of karma:

1. **Sanchita karma** is the sum total of all accumulated past actions in all of our previous individual lifetimes.
2. **Prarabdha karma** is that portion of Sanchita karma which has resulted in this present birth. As such, it is the kind of karma most of us are concerned with from day to day. Included in this type of karma is the position of the planets at the moment of our birth. It is upon this category of karma that astrology is based.

   Prarabdha karma is the one kind of karma that cannot be directly changed. After all, it is impossible to go back in time and change the position of the planets at the time of our birth. Thus, each of us has an astrological karmic blueprint that is as precise in its way as our DNA.

   But the working out of this type of karma *can* be changed. Although we cannot change the position of the planets at the time of our birth, we can change the way we receive those influences or vibrations. As discussed in chapter 2, the practice of mantra changes our inner conditions so that when the vibrations reach us, the effects are different than they would have been if we had not changed our inner landscape.

3. **Agami karma** results from our present willful actions in this life, which will, of course, have an effect on future returning karma.

4. **Kriyamana karma** results immediately from our present actions.

Changing the Effects of Karma

Sanchita karma, Kriyamana karma, and Agami karma can all be positively affected in our current lifetime through conscious decisions. Prarabdha karma, however, is defined at the moment of our birth. That karma will be ours through this entire lifetime.

Although you cannot change the position of the planets at the time of your birth, you can affect your Prarabdha karma. You can change the way you receive the influences or vibrations of the planets you were "born under." To illustrate this point, the American spiritual teacher Donald Walters—also known for years as Swami Kriyananda—created a wonderful analogy. It may be "in our planets," Walters said, "that when a specific moment arrives we will fall down a flight of stairs and break a leg. But this need not be. We can prepare ourselves spiritually, so that when that moment arrives, all we do is stub our toe."

This is a powerful concept. The stars' influence upon us can indeed be modified by the state in which we receive those mysterious vibrations. But how can we make such inner changes? How can we change ourselves so that when that particular moment with its inherent propensities arrives, we only "stub our toe"?

Changing the Inner Landscape

The work we do with mantra is governed by Agami karma. Using a mantra is an action in the present that will affect our future karma. When we practice mantra, our inner conditions change so that when the vibrations reach us, the effects are different from what they would have been if we had not changed our inner landscape. Additionally, the work that takes place with mantra now becomes part of our Agami karma in a positive sense. Our previous free-will actions have now come to our aid. And since we are affecting our present good for the better, we are also working with Kriyamana karma.

Chanting mantras, then, works directly with each type of karma and helps us overcome unfavorable conditions we may have inadvertently or ignorantly created in this or some other life. How, exactly, can this take place?

As we work with the sound vibrations of mantra, those vibrations change our inner physical and etheric condition. When a particular mantra has been used over a period of time, the physical body, the chakras, and all elements of the subtle body become tuned in a slightly different manner.

Karma can be likened to seeds that have first been stored, and eventually planted. When the right conditions are at last present, the seeds of karma sprout. The purpose of karma reduction or elimination, then, is to destroy the seeds. By diligent practice of Sanskrit mantra we burn the seeds of bad karma created by past deeds and past states of mind.

Consider, for example, a mantra for eliminating anger. The elimination of anger through mantra involves changing the vibration of where certain patterns are stored in the physical and subtle bodies. Anger is stored in specific organs and sections of the body. While the exact location may vary from individual to individual, the storage place in each of us is quite specific. When some outer condition has an effect upon the place or places where patterns of anger-energy are stored, we become angry.

The planets can be thought of as "triggers" that activate certain inner tendencies. When the planets pass through certain astrological signs or alignments that resonate with our astrological DNA, as represented by our natal chart, the stored patterns also begin to resonate. Thus, we may become angry through an event that normally might not produce that effect. The personality goes along with the inner activation of the patterns and we react to some incident with anger. Although it is true that we tend to be made angry by the same kinds of stimuli, it is also true that planetary movement can cause new patterns to appear.

The use of mantra with the conscious intention of eliminating anger will begin a process whereby those patterns break down and the stored energy becomes transmuted and available for other purposes.

In psychology there is a saying: "Find your anger and there you will find great energy." By redirecting hostility, you can become more capable and productive. The ancient spiritual teachings completely agree with this modern idea.

Astrological activity can also produce positive effects. The unexpected offer of a great job, meeting the person of our dreams, and winning the lottery are all examples of positive karma at work. The idea of balance then enters the picture. We want to optimize positive karma, minimize negative karma, and have the understanding to tell the difference between the two. In undertaking the use of mantra to achieve the proper karmic balance, it is also useful to pray for wisdom.

What Frequency Is My Spleen, Please?

Each organ in the physical body has a specific vibration. This vibration is its natural state. If you imagine that all of humanity's livers, for instance, vibrate within a small, general frequency range in their natural state, you have the right idea. Now here come the complications. All actions have consequences and repercussions, whether the act is conscious or unconscious. These consequences are impossible for us to see, by and large, because the effects are simultaneously subatomic and grandly universal. And these consequences give rise to biological effects on the body. The change may not be immediately visible or even manifest in the life where it was created. But it will manifest sooner or later unless the energy is transmuted.

Please remember the following:

- *Matter and energy can be neither created nor destroyed* (though they can be reorganized). In modern physics this is the First Law of Thermodynamics.
- *All things return to their source.* This is a statement of the Law of Karma.
- *As ye sow, so shall ye reap.* This biblical injunction states the Law of Karma metaphorically.

While we may know similar phrases by the dozen, we may not believe that we can do anything about these forces and their effects on our lives. But mantra can sometimes help transmute the karma of this life and our many previous lives.

If there has been a prolonged bad karma over several lifetimes, it may be difficult to use mantra to change the health of an organ in one lifetime. Then the soul may choose to take drastic action and clear the slate all at once with cancer or some other catastrophic condition that burns up all of the negative vibrations in a single lifetime. However, people sometimes draw on their good karma to counteract the negative karma of disease, and a miraculous recovery takes place.

Astrological Primer

Each part of the body is ruled by a specific astrological sign. For example, the heart and spine are ruled by Leo. The arms and lungs are controlled by Gemini. Reproduction and elimination are in Scorpio's domain. On pages 96–97 is a table, "The Planets and Our Bodies," which will serve as a quick reference. (If you desire a more detailed analysis, astrologer Jeff Mayo has written several books covering this material in depth.)

Each astrological sign has a planet that generally wields and directs its energy in our local universe. For example, Capricorn: Saturn; Scorpio: Mars; Leo: the Sun. The effects of a variety of karmically related events will be different for each person in each sign. In addition, we are all influenced by a ruling of twelve influencing "houses," as they are called, which rotate around each person's chart. The list of astrological signs and the planets presented later in this chapter shows these correspondences.

For everyone who attains the ages of twenty-nine, fifty-eight, and eighty-six, the planet Saturn returns to the exact location it occupied at his or her birth, and a new learning cycle begins. Many astrologers refer to this period as the Saturn Return. Often called the planet of lessons, Saturn begins to present new categories of lessons to each of us when it returns to its place in our natal birth chart.

When I was in my late twenties, the strategies I had developed for success in life stopped working. I was forced, over a period of several years, to change my entirely materialistic view of life into one based upon a spiritual view of things. I was completely confounded by new kinds of events in my life that were decidedly unpleasant, and for which I was completely unprepared.

The difficulties persisted until I met someone who told me that I was now in my Saturn period. I was given a mantra for the planet Saturn to help alleviate my problems. I undertook the repetition of this mantra, and within a few short weeks things began to change dramatically for the better even though I was still within my Saturn period. More important, because I *knew* I was in for some difficulties, and *had* to go through them, I could accept more calmly that I needed to face certain changes. I could choose the way I responded to inevitable problems with the help of mantra.

Astrological Approaches

There is an Eastern approach and a Western approach to astrology, and they both work. One is lunar-based and the other is solar-based. But the position of the planets remains the same for both systems. Therefore, for the purpose of work upon your planetary karma, it does not matter which system you employ.

If you have not already done so, it is a good idea to have your natal chart done. Any competent astrologer can readily tell you the easy and difficult aspects within your natal chart. You may have difficult aspects involving one planet or another. Conversely, you undoubtedly also have things in your life that are very easy. The planets can teach us many lessons.

The Planets and Our Bodies

Any astrologer or book on astrology will tell you that certain parts of the body are governed by specific planetary principles. For example, the knees, spleen, and skeletal system are under strong influence of the planet Saturn. In astrology they say that these parts of the body are "governed" by the Saturn principle. Here is how various organs are related to celestial bodies, along with a mantra related to the planet or other celestial body with the greatest influence on that body part.

Heart, spine, diaphragm, thymus, blood, and veins	Sun	*Om Sri Suryaya Namaha*
Stomach including gastric processes, breasts, lymphatic and other nonblood fluid systems such as perspiration and saliva, sympathetic nervous system	Moon	*Om Sri Chandraya Namaha*
Hands, arms, lungs, sensory organs, some thyroid gland influence	Mercury	*Om Sri Budhaya Namaha*
Throat, neck, kidneys, secondary connection with sex organs and feet, some thyroid gland influence	Venus	*Om Sri Shukraya Namaha*
Sex organs, adrenal glands, red blood cells	Mars	*Om Sri Angarakaya Namaha*
Liver, gallbladder, posterior lobe of the pituitary (related to growth), thighs	Jupiter	*Om Sri Gurave Namaha*

| Spleen, skeletal system including cartilage, skin, lower leg from the knee to the ankle, anterior lobe of the pituitary gland (related to body type) | Saturn | *Om Sri Shanaishwaraya Swaha* |

In Eastern, lunar-based astrology, a person may be said to enter a Mars period lasting seven years. Things in life may become difficult for no apparent reason. A Vedic astrologer (they are not that easy to find) can easily spot these and other periods of potential problems in relationships, business, and the like. Knowing which planetary aspects may be causing problems offers a route to clearing them.

For instance, Samantha's mother was bothered for years by rheumatoid arthritis. She had trouble getting around and was housebound most days of the week. When Samantha spoke to me about her mother's problem, the first thing that popped into my mind was the planetary energy that rules the skeletal system: Saturn. Perhaps working with the energy of the planet could help "soften" the influence of the energy of Saturn and alleviate the mother's condition. Saturn also has powerful connection to the knees, lower leg from the knee to the ankle, and the spleen. I explained the rationale and the associated mantra to Samantha, who later told me that her mother was saying her Saturn mantra regularly and getting around much better.

Om Sri Shanaishwaraya Swaha

(OM SHREE SHAHN-EHSH-WAHR-EYE-YAH SWAH-HA)

"Om and salutations to Saturn, the planet of lessons."

The Power of the Astrological Sign

The planetary alignments in our individual birth charts can present unique problems and lessons for each of us. Most astrologers who interpret your birth chart will discuss the "easy" and the "difficult" of your planets by their relationship to other planets. Usually they do not know of any way for you to ease difficult alignments. But through the use of Sanskrit mantras for individual planets, you *can* change your planetary karma. Here is a list of astrological signs and the planets and karmic bodies that rule them, as well as the mantras associated with each celestial body, including Rahu and Ketu, the karmic nodes of the moon.

Aries	Mars	*Om Sri Angarakaya Namaha*
Taurus	Venus	*Om Sri Shukraya Namaha*
Gemini	Mercury	*Om Sri Budhaya Namaha*
Cancer	Moon	*Om Sri Chandraya Namaha*
Leo	Sun	*Om Sri Suryaya Namaha*
Virgo	Mercury	*Om Sri Budhaya Namaha*
Libra	Venus	*Om Sri Shukraya Namaha*
Scorpio	Mars/Pluto	*Om Sri Angarakaya Namaha*
Sagittarius	Jupiter	*Om Sri Gurave Namaha*
Capricorn	Saturn	*Om Sri Shanaishwaraya Namaha*
Aquarius	Uranus/Saturn	*Om Sri Shanaishwaraya Namaha*
Pisces	Jupiter/Neptune	*Om Sri Gurave Namaha*
Dragon's Head	North Node of Moon	*Om Sri Rahuve Namaha*
Dragon's Tail	South Node of Moon	*Om Sri Ketuve Namaha*

Working with Planetary Energies

Once you have the information contained in your natal chart, you can begin working on your life with a clear idea of where to start. The Sanskrit mantras below translate roughly to "Salutations to the presiding spirit of the planet————." The Vedas teach that everything has consciousness within it. They also say that planets and stars are conscious in a way that is completely different from the way in which we humans are conscious.

Below are short forms of mantras for seven planets and the karmic nodes of the moon. If you are having difficulty in some part of your life, find the planetary mantra that seems to come closest to it and work with that mantra. If you really want to roll up your sleeves, work with the mantra for forty consecutive days.

Sometimes there seems to be more than one planet involved. This can be true because of a shared aspect between them, or because of two unrelated planetary positions. In the latter case, work with both planetary mantras. This can be done either sequentially (forty days of one, followed by forty days of the other) or by working with both for a period each day. Follow whichever of these strategies feels better to you.

Short Planetary Mantras

Sun   *Om Suryaya Namaha*
         (Om Soor-yah-yah Nahm-ah-ha)
         "Om and salutations to Surya, presiding spirit of the Sun."

Moon   *Om Chandraya Namaha*
         (Om Chahn-drah-yah Nahm-ah-ha)
         "Om and salutations to Chandra, presiding spirit of the Moon."

Mars   *Om Angarakaya Namaha*
         (Om Ahng-gah-rah-kah-ya Nahm-ah-ha)
         "Om and salutations to the presiding spirit of the planet Mars."

Mercury *Om Budhaya Namaha*
         (Om Bood-hah-yah Nahm-ah-ha)
         "Om and salutations to Buddha, presiding spirit of the planet
         Mercury."

Jupiter *Om Gurave Namaha*
         (Om Goo-rah-vey Nahm-ah-ha)
         "Om and salutations to Guru, presiding spirit of the planet
         Jupiter."

Venus   *Om Shukraya Namaha*
             (Om Shoo-krah-yah Nahm-ah-ha)
             "Om and salutations to Shukra, presiding spirit of the planet
             Venus."

Saturn   *Om Shanaishcharaya Namaha*
             (Om Shahn-eish-chahr-eye-yah Nahm-ah-ha)
             The ending of the Sanskrit word for the planet Saturn, "Shani,"
             changes endings depending upon the use of Namaha (neutral
             ending) or Swaha (feminine ending). Thus, for the mantra
             ending with "namaha" the mantra is "Om Sri Shanaishcharaya
             Namaha" but for the "swaha" ending the mantra is "Om Sri
             Shanaishwaraya Swaha."
             Om Shanaishwaraya Swaha
             (Om Shahn-eish-wahr-eye-yah Swa-ha)
             "Om and salutations to Shani, presiding spirit of the planet
             Saturn."
             When the energy of the body rises to the solar plexus, as it does at
             age twenty-nine, the addition of "Sri" to the mantra aids the work
             of the mantra. The ending then changes from "namaha" to "swaha."

Rahu   *Om Rahuve Namaha*
             (Om Rah-hoo-vey Nahm-ah-ha)
             "Om and salutations to Rahu, presiding spirit of the North Node
             of the Moon."

Ketu   *Om Ketuve Namaha*
             (Om Key-too-vey Nahm-ah-ha)
             "Om and salutations to Ketu, presiding spirit of the South Node
             of the Moon."

Movement of Energy Centers as We Grow

When we are young, our general energy center stays in the first chakra
area. We are in the process of developing our personality and a way of
dealing with the world. Socialization and myriad other person-forming
activities take place up to the age of twelve or thirteen.

When we begin to awaken sexually, the general energy center rises to the second chakra area. Puberty is an extremely stressful time because we are literally forced out of our old way of being and thrust into a new one. When sexuality appears there are new rules we must learn that seem to appear out of nowhere. There are completely different methods of behavior to be developed, for instance, toward others of the same sex and the opposite sex. Everyone understands this.

When we are roughly twenty-eight years old, another new cycle begins. The energy center rises to the third chakra area. Again we become interested in life in new ways. The rules change once more, but more subtly. Suddenly our career can seem much more important than it did before. The alarm on the biological clock can go off, creating a tremendous urge to procreate. Competition in life often takes on a whole new level of importance. And the changes in life all seem to accelerate. Why should this be?

Sociological and psychological statistics concerning young adults show that between the ages of twenty-eight and thirty-five the greatest number of significant life changes take place. For instance, single individuals marry more during this period than during any other seven-year period of life. Conversely, the highest number of married couples divorce during this age span than in any other. These ages also show the highest incidence of job change and career path change and the highest incidence of schizophrenia. The list goes on and on. Significant figures on young adults kept by sociologists and psychologists support what astrologers have been saying for centuries. This period is a time of great change. It is a time when we truly begin our adult life. When we reach the second Saturn cycle at age fifty-eight, the process occurs again with a new set of lessons. These can be change-of-life lessons, mature-relationship lessons, health lessons, and so forth. Anytime Saturn returns to the same position in its orbit that it occupied when you were born, a new learning cycle is triggered.

So if you are in this Saturn period in your life, or you know someone who is, there is something that can make the journey through it easier. The mantra of the planet Saturn can be a tremendous help.

Saturn's Lessons

Saturn is the planet of lessons, and it works in a very specific way to "trigger" karma. Staying approximately two and one-half years in each astrological sign, Saturn energy activates certain parts of our karma as it enters each sign. We are presented with new things we should try to learn or master. The Saturn mantra can help us more quickly understand what those lessons might be and move on. Although most astrologers will tell you that the lesson of Saturn can be difficult, there have been cases where the influence of Saturn has been helpful and beneficial simply because the person has learned and assimilated the pertinent lesson.

For instance, if you have previously learned some lesson with regard to employment, you may find that the movement of Saturn into a new sign triggers a fantastic new job offer from a completely unexpected quarter. In such an instance, Saturn acts as a positive trigger to release this unexpected windfall. If there were lessons to be learned, the trigger effect of Saturn might release something less pleasant.

I once got a teaching position when Saturn entered Leo. This is supposed to be a terrible position for Saturn, particularly for someone like me who has the Moon in Leo. But instead, I applied for (not thinking I had a prayer) and secured a full-time teaching position at a university in Washington, D.C. It is true I was hired to teach broadcasting, where I had good professional credentials. But I had no Ph.D., which is almost a prerequisite for a full-time position. I concluded that I must have assimilated whatever lessons were needed for "teaching" long ago. Although I was very grateful to God for this blessing, it was not lost on me that karma, very good karma in this case, was involved. Saturn, usually thought of as the deliverer of unsettling lessons of one sort or another, had given me a gift because I had already learned the lessons involved.

To gain maximum benefit from the Saturn mantra, say the short form at least 25,000 times each time Saturn changes the sign it moves through.

Om Sri Shanaishwaraya Swaha

(OM SHREE SHAHN-EHSH-WAHR-EYE-YAH SWAH-HA)

Repeating this mantra 108 times takes about five minutes if you say it neither too fast nor too slowly. This means that approximately 2,000 per hour are completed at this rate. This calculates out to twelve and one-half hours to complete the 25,000. This means that if you repeated the Saturn mantra for ten minutes each day, you would reach 25,000 in about 115 days—one-third of a year. This can be completed easily just driving in your car from one place to another. Or, while riding the subway, repeating it to yourself mentally.

Not to overstate things, Saturn mantra repetition is highly recommended for smoothing your path in life by helping you understand the lessons you have set for yourself through Prarabdha karma: the position of the planets at the time of your birth.

Similarly, if a Vedic astrologer tells you that you are entering a difficult Mars period, then work with *Om Angarakaya Namaha* to help clear the way you receive those vibrations, and you will notice an improvement.

You can change your karma. There are people all over the planet doing it every day through repetition of Sanskrit mantra. The idea of changing karma and reducing karma is the entire point of most spiritual disciplines. However, by utilizing Sanskrit mantras for specific planets, you can focus your efforts on an area of your life or condition that may be particularly bothersome.

An Early Warning System

In 1973 I got a new job with a public television channel in northern Virginia as an associate producer for children's programs. On my starting day for the job I got up, dressed, ate, and prepared to leave. I got as far as opening the door and was greeted immediately by the shrieking of a crow. It was seated on the fork of two branches of a tree not fifteen feet from my front door. The crow was looking directly at me and screeching at the top of its little lungs. It was unsettling, to put it mildly.

I closed the door and tried to stop my heart from racing. I opened the door again and the same crow screeched at me again. When I closed the door it became silent. I sat down on a nearby chair. I tried to think of everything I knew about crows. Unfortunately, I knew almost nothing about crows. But I did recall that in Carlos Castaneda's second book, *A Separate Reality,* crows were said to indicate the presence of sorcerers. Oh, swell. What a comfort.

The third time I opened the door, the crow was gone. I went on my way to work and had about as bad a first day as one can have on a job. I didn't know whether I would last there or not. Everything began to settle down the next day, and after several weeks the job turned out quite well. That was my introduction to crows.

Over the next few weeks I underwent a course I call Crows 101. I quickly learned that anytime I would see or hear a crow, an unpleasant incident or situation would ensue within the next one to fifteen minutes. It became axiomatic. Almost hit by a car while walking along the road. Missed my bus by thirty seconds. Accosted by some loony stranger for no apparent reason I could figure out. Lost my keys. Rammed with a shopping cart while in line at the supermarket minding my own business. Every one of these incidents was preceded by the screeching of a crow somewhere close to me until I paid attention.

It got to the point that when I saw a crow or heard one cawing, I would begin to cringe, wondering what would happen next. It wasn't as if I could tell anyone. I know because I tried. After I attempted to tell one of my housemates about the whole thing with the crows, he either humored me or avoided me as much as possible. My stories must have seemed quite odd to other people, so I soon shut up about the crows and endured them as a new harbinger of gloom.

Two months later, I gathered enough nerve to tell a spiritual teacher about my "thing" with the crows on the off chance that something might come of it. Nodding, the teacher indicated that the crow was the symbol in nature for the planet Saturn. He inquired about my age. I was in my early thirties at the time. The teacher said I was nearing the end of my Saturn Return and gave me the mantra *Om Sri Shanaishwaraya Swaha* to work with, explaining that it related to the energy of the planet Saturn.

I worked with that mantra for several hours every day. Within a few days, I began to notice changes. And I found that my attention was being drawn to what the crow was doing.

Crows do all sorts of things, I discovered. Sometimes the crow would be looking at its feet. Sometimes it would be stretching its wings in a most peculiar manner. It would do strange things with its beak. It could make strange little vocal clicking sounds. It would sometimes appear to be staring at its own navel. I paid as much attention as I could and tried some experiments.

In just two weeks, I found that I could see a crow doing something, change my course of action, and avoid an unpleasant experience. I continued to work with the mantra and all the difficulties subsided after about forty days.

Over the years I have continued to work off and on with that mantra. I renew it every once in a while. Crows are now part of the way I relate to life. They have become a very friendly "early warning sign" that I now view as a gift. There have been instances when I would be speeding on the freeway and a crow would wheel in front of me. I instinctively knew that this meant there was a radar trap or police car coming up. Now, whenever I am driving and see a crow, I slow down and become very cautious. Invariably a police car will glide into view, lurking in the far right lane waiting for unsuspecting speeders like myself. Or I will round a freeway underpass and spot a radar trap. I have avoided many tickets and accidents with the help of the crows.

The crows have become such a part of my life that I shared them with my friend Michael Weir. This spiritual man at first showed just the slightest skepticism, but agreed to look out for them. A couple of weeks later he returned to me with his own breathless tales of what the crows had warned him about.

A Word about Namaha and Swaha

Namaha means "I offer." There are many ways to express the idea of offering. Namaha is neither masculine nor feminine. It is gender neutral. Parsing the energy contained in the word *Namaha* you get something like this: *Nam* produces a certain quality of energy in the base center, genital center, and heart center. *Ah* produces energy in the heart and throat. *Ha* produces energy in one side of the two-sided brow center where the masculine and feminine currents meet. Intent also colors the energy: *Nam* means "name," as in "divine word." *Maha* means "great." Together, *Namaha* means "the foregoing is a great name for the principle used in the mantra that I now offer."

Swaha is a feminine ending that means "I offer to the higher realms." *Swaha Loka* is "realm of the Sun." But it is also used to connote those realms which lie beyond the Sun or solar region. So the use of *Swaha* is determined somewhat by its context. In one context it may clearly refer to the solar region, while in another it may refer to realms that lie beyond. For general purposes, *Swaha* is used as a mantra ending if you are twenty-nine years of age or older, except when otherwise indicated by the explanations for certain mantras in this book.

Gifts of the Sun

Professional astrologers often use the analogy of a building to describe the workings of the Sun sign, the Moon sign, and the rising sign—the "big three" portions of a natal chart. If you build a building, the superstructure, girders, power plant, heating, and air-conditioning all correspond to the Sun sign. The way the building looks both inside and outside, including the facade composed of wood, brick, stucco, or other finishing, as well as the decoration of the inner rooms, corresponds to the Moon sign. The outer look of the building is our personality and the decoration of the inner rooms is the way we construct our relationships in life, both personal and professional. The reason the building was built corresponds to the rising sign: why we came here to the Earth.

Everything starts from the basic Sun sign. It is the placement of the Sun in the various signs that gives our internal power plant certain characteristics. Since the Sun is the power source from which all springs, it is not surprising that there are a number of mantras that work to produce specific conditions affecting our power plant. The solar mantras given here are said to produce certain effects, the "fruit" of the mantra. As you repeat the mantra, a certain portion of its power will become evident. This is called mantra siddhi, the power of the mantra.

Siddhi is a general term for spiritual power or ability. Therefore, some power or ability deriving from the saying of the mantra should become evident.

The generally accepted time for achieving mantra siddhi is universally given in texts and references as a minimum of 125,000 repetitions. To achieve the fruit of these solar mantras, therefore, a minimum of 125,000 repetitions is prescribed. For a short mantra like *Om Suryaya Namaha*, it is fairly easy to repeat the mantra, say, 2,000 times per hour. At this rate, it would take sixty-two and one-half hours to complete 125,000 repetitions. This could easily be accomplished in forty days. Chapter 3 contains a more detailed discussion of a forty-day discipline.

Short mantras lend themselves easily to a forty-day discipline. Driving on the highway or riding the subway provides a great opportunity to work with mantras and it is much cheaper than talking on a cell phone.

Sun Mantras and Their Fruit

Om Mitraya Namaha	Light of Universal Friendship
Om Ravaye Namaha	Light of Compelling Radiance
Om Suryaya Namaha	Dispeller of Darkness or Ignorance

Om Bhanave Namaha	Shining Principle
Om Khagaya Namaha	All-Pervading Light
Om Pushne Namaha	Light of Mystic Fire
Om Hiranyagarbhaya Namaha	Golden-Colored One: healing gold
Om Marichaye Namaha	Light: obvious and subtle, as at dawn and dusk
Om Adityaya Namaha	Light of the Sage: an aspect of Vishnu
Om Savitre Namaha	Light of Enlightenment
Om Arkaya Namaha	Light That Removes Afflictions
Om Bhaskaraya Namaha	Brilliance: the light of intelligence

As you read the list above, perhaps one example of the fruit may make a sudden, strong impression. This indicates that some part of you wants or needs this principle of solar and spiritual light.

Rising and Moon Signs

If you are concerned about the movement of planets over your Moon sign or your rising sign in the astrological chart, consult one of the previously listed charts, find the mantra for the planetary energy that concerns you, and complete 25,000 repetitions.

Taking Charge

Each planet acts as a trigger in our astrological makeup in a different way. But the mantras related to the planets can clear up difficulties just as a powerful solvent cuts through grease. Knowledge, it is said, is power. Knowing that there is a powerful connection between our karma, our health, and the orderly movement of the planets through the heavens is a first step in minimizing difficulties. Putting mantra into practice turns that knowledge into usable power.

7

Mantras and Health

Health problems are part of the human condition. We have all had physical maladies which we would have tried to heal ourselves, if only we had known what to do. Even modern medical science, with its antibiotics and flu shots, has made only limited progress in addressing many common health issues.

This chapter does not offer a panacea. Mantra is not a cure for all ills. But mantras can dramatically contribute to our overall health and well-being, and as with all life challenges, the more tools you have to work with, the better your chances for a long and productive life.

Note that most healing mantras are general in nature. You will not find a specific mantra for every health problem, although in the preceding chapter I did discuss mantras for specific areas of the body. Most of the formulas presented here can be applied to almost any condition. Whatever mantra you finally select, be open to looking at all methods of healing the condition that may appear.

Be Open-minded and Be Ready

I once knew a man who practiced mantra to relieve the debilitating condition called chronic fatigue syndrome, or CFS. He was diligent and focused in his efforts. One day, after he had been working to improve his condition through mantra for nearly a month, he had a visitor whom he had not seen for some time. As they talked, the visitor asked the man about his health problem. When the man mentioned CFS, the visitor excitedly declared that he had recently come across an article in the May 1990 issue of the British medical journal *Lancet*. The article reported on research that verified the efficacy of a fairly simple course of treatment for CFS. The visitor urged him to read the article and then try the treatment. The man scoffed and waved him away. The visitor went so far as to tell him about a local woman he knew who had tried the treatment and improved substantially over a six-week period, after having struggled with CFS for four years. Still the man would not listen. He was waiting for a miracle. Of course the miracle had already come, but he had missed it entirely.

Those practicing Sanskrit mantra for healing purposes must not abandon all other routes to healing. The result of your mantra discipline may not be what you expect. Be open and ready to take any route to recovery, even an unexpected one.

When we work with mantra we are working with energy, and energy is never lost. It will appear in some way. But we must not attempt to dictate through belief systems just how that energy will work.

As you look over the healing mantras presented in the next pages, please understand that if you undertake a discipline of any of these mantras, you will be setting certain forces in motion. The energy itself will work in a specific way. Your intention will add focus and power to the practice. But you must also be ready to receive a result when the time comes.

Fibromyalgia Healing Success

Cynthia estimates that she had fibromyalgia for about twenty years. At first she was completely disabled by the ailment, which is characterized by inflamed and aching joints. Nobody, including doctors, could tell her what was wrong with her. People came to think her problem was psychological. Doing her best to cope, Cynthia took undemanding part-time jobs to make a living, while feeling rotten most of the time.

I didn't know any of this when Cynthia enrolled in my class. After the first class meeting, she stayed until everyone else had left. She asked if I had ever heard of fibromyalgia, and I said I was quite familiar with it. When she asked if I knew of something that might help her, I gave her two mantras to practice, the first for the spleen, the second to remove energy blockages.

Om Sri Shanaishwaraya Swaha (for the spleen)

(OM SHREE SHAHN-EHSH-WAHR-EYE-YAH SWAH-HA)

Om Gum Ganapatayei Namaha (to remove energy blockages)

(OM GUM GUH-NUH-PUH-TUH-YEI NAHM-AH-HA)

I also gave her a long Rama healing mantra, which I will present later in this chapter.

Finally, I recommended that she start a meditative but energetic yogic breathing exercise, pranayama, or alternate nostril breathing. I could see that her life energy, or prana, was diffuse and scattered. After some instruction, she started the breathing practice right then and there.

Instructions for Alternate Nostril Pranayama Breathing.
There are endless varieties taught for this simple breathing exercise. Each teacher seems to have a slightly different method for the practice, including counting the number of seconds one breathes in, holds the breath, and exhales. However, what follows is the very simplest method for performing the practice that was taught by Swami Sivananda in Rishikesh, India, for forty years. It simply involves breathing in the precise manner given here, without the need for measuring the seconds for breathing in, holding the breath, or breathing out.

Prepare yourself to sit quietly for a minimum of five minutes and a maximum of fifteen minutes. Holding your right thumb against your right nostril to close it off, inhale deeply through your left nostril until the lungs are full to capacity without strain. Now using the middle finger of your right hand to close the left nostril, breathe out through the left nostril. Once the lungs have expelled the air, breathe in through the same nostril, the left, that you just breathed in. This is one alternate nostril breath. Perform this four more times for a total of five alternate nostril breaths. Now rest for thirty seconds or so, then perform five more alternate nostril breaths. Rest again and repeat the process a third time. Once you have finished, you have performed three "rounds" of five alternate nostril breaths. As you grow in proficiency, you can do ten, fifteen, twenty, or more breaths in a round.

This technique is both calming and energizing, balancing the energies of both sides of your mind and body.

After just one week, Cynthia had a new glow about her. She smiled sheepishly in the next class and said that she was already starting to feel better. After six weeks, her whole demeanor had changed. She was charged with energy and confidence. Three months later, she indicated that she was still taking it a bit easy if she started to get tired, but that she felt completely cured. She subsequently had a profound private meditation experience that, for her, confirmed that she was now completely recovered from fibromyalgia.

The Celestial Physician

The science of healing is as old as humanity. Shamans and medicine men and women have existed in every culture. Sometimes the very valuable esoteric knowledge of healing herbs and plants is passed down through generations. The ancient Vedic records include detailed histories of shamans or medicine people. One such healer in the Hindu tradition was called Dhanvantre, "the celestial physician." His mantra is used to find a path to the appropriate healing method for any health problem.

Om Sri Dhanvantre Namaha

(OM SHREE DON-VON-TREY NAHM-AH-HA)

"Salutations to the being and power of the Celestial Physician."

In traditional households in southern India, women chant this mantra as they prepare food to infuse it with the powerful healing vibrations that ward off disease. In other households the mantra is chanted during preparation of food for the sick or infirm.

You can chant this mantra while concentrating upon any condition that you would like remedied or healed. Chant it for at least 12,500 times, then be open to the manner in which healing may manifest. Remember that healing may be achieved according to traditional medicine, or through some other means altogether. Be open-minded and do not hold expectations of how the healing will occur.

Rochelle's Story

For several weeks Rochelle had been having stomach problems caused by nervousness. When her doctors seemed unable to help her, Rochelle called me to ask if there was a mantra that could help her stomach. After a brief meditation, I determined that the Dhanvantre could be of benefit. She began repeating it every day, and after just a short time began to feel better. She kept on with the mantra even after her problems had disappeared, to ensure that she wouldn't relapse.

After several weeks of practice, Rochelle had to drive her husband to the airport for an unexpected business trip. Because of other conditions in her life at the time, this was very unsettling for her. After she had dropped her husband off at the airport and was driving home, she had a panic attack. Without even thinking, she reflexively began to chant *Om Sri Dhanvantre Namaha*. After only half-a-dozen repetitions, the attack subsided. A bit shaken but otherwise feeling normal, she drove home without further difficulty. She was amazed at how this mantra had calmed her anxiety in only a few moments. She now feels that she has control over her nervous stomach condition, even under stressful conditions.

In using any mantra, it's important to plan your discipline and monitor the results. These procedures were discussed in chapter 3, "How to Use Your Mantra." Here is a brief refresher:

Place.
Set aside a place where you will practice the mantra discipline every day.

Time of Day.
Schedule a specific time, either once or twice a day, when you will sit for your discipline. Some people have very busy schedules and once a day is all they can allow themselves. Others with more flexible schedules can easily manage once in the morning and once in the evening.

Number of Repetitions.
You may decide to accomplish 108, or 200, or more repetitions of your selected mantra while sitting in your special place. Also remember that you may do the mantra informally at other times and places throughout the day.

After you have decided on the particulars of your discipline, fix your starting and ending date. If helpful, place a calendar near your meditation spot with the dates clearly marked.

Other General Healing Mantras

In addition to the Dhanvantre mantra, there are other general healing mantras that you can apply with good results. Here are some of them.

Water Mantra.

Water has been used for mystical ceremonies and healing ceremonies for as long as humans have lived in communities. Here is a mantra which proclaims that ordinary water, when charged with God's healing power, can do the job.

Oushadhim Jahnavi Toyam Vaidyo Narayana Harihi

(OW-SHAH-DEEM JAH-NAH-VEE TOH-YUHM
VEYED-YOH NAH-RAH-YAH-NAH HA-REE-HEE)

*"Water touched by the Spirit of God is the best
medicine, because God is the best doctor."*

There are powerful chakras in the hands that are open in many hands-on healers. If you think your hand chakras are open and functioning even a little, you can chant this mantra while holding your palm over a cup or glass of water. In this way you are not only asking that the Holy Spirit work through you and this water to promote healing, but you are also pouring healing prana from your hand into the water, which will then be consumed.

General Healing Power of the Sun (Inner and Outer).

In chapter 6 the use of solar and planetary mantras for alleviating distressful conditions was discussed. For now, know that the use of the mantra given below activates certain petals in the solar plexus chakra which then begin to produce powerful healing vibrations. This mantra can also be chanted at the Sun, asking that Great Sun Being to send forth the Arkaya energy (that which heals afflictions) or the Hiranyagarbha energy (that which heals with the golden-colored rays) to heal the one afflicted. When using these mantras it is beneficial for the sick person to spend some time in the sun every day.

Om Arkaya Namaha

(OM AHR-KAH-YAH NAHM-AH-HA)

*"Om and salutations to the Shining
One who removes afflictions."*

Om Hiranyagarbhaya Namaha

(OM HERE-AHN-YAH-GAHR-BAH-YAH NAHM-AH-HA)

*"Om and salutations to the Shining One
who heals and is golden-colored."*

Sun Mantras for Healing of the Eyes.
The power of the Sun can also be invoked to heal the eyes. As above, chant the following mantra to the Sun, and try to get the sick or injured person some exposure to the Sun each day.

Om Grinihi Suryaya Adityom

(OM GRIH-NEE-HEE SOOR-YAH-YAH AH-DEET-YOHM)

"Om and salutations to the Shining One who heals the eyes."

Kay called me one day with some sad news. She had been to the doctor because her eyes had been bothering her. When the results of the tests came in, they revealed a degenerative eye condition for which surgery would be needed. It was scheduled some seven weeks in the future.

Kay was upset because even with the surgery the doctors were not very optimistic. She asked for help. I gave her the above mantra to do and we scheduled a healing ceremony, or puja, at the conclusion of her efforts. She decided to do the classical forty-day spiritual discipline.

For forty days she did the mantra morning and evening. When she had time, she would also do it in between those meditations by taking short breaks throughout her day. After she had concluded her forty-day discipline, we performed the ceremony with a group of friends in attendance. The fifteen of us had a wonderful time as we conducted the ancient ceremony.

The very next week, Kay went to the doctor for a presurgery examination. When she returned home she called me breathlessly to report that her condition had stopped progressing. The doctor had found that there had been no further degeneration at all and things actually seemed a little better. He decided to postpone the surgery until things should get worse again. It has been three years as of this writing, and the surgery is still on hold. Kay is still fine, and checks in regularly with her physician.

Mantras for Eye and Lung Conditions.

There is a pair of celestial healers called the Ashwini devatas. They have responsibility for protecting the inward and outward breath and the eyes. For the lungs, invoking them strengthens the breathing. For the eyes, dimness of the appearance of objects can be helped. In employing these mantras, use the previously discussed methods of determining the time and place of discipline.

Om Ashwina Tejasa Chakshuhu

(OM AHSH-WEEN-AH TEH-JAH-SAH CHAHK-SHOO-HOO)

*"Om and salutations to the Ashwini devatas
who heal the eyes and keep them bright."*

Om Ashwina Bheshajam
Madhu Bheshajam

(OM AHSH-WEEN-AH BEH-SHAH-JAHM
MAH-DOO BEH-SHAH-JAHM)

*"Om and salutations to the Ashwina devatas.
Kindly bless us with the honey of your healing balm."*

If you have a condition that you feel would be helped by either of these mantras, complete a forty-day discipline in the classical manner discussed in chapter 3.

Healing with Rama Mantras

In the Old and New Testaments of the Bible, we find magnificent spiritual figures with great gifts that may be offered to deserving ones. We also find spiritual authority in the form of speaking a thing and making it so. Jesus said, "Heaven and earth may pass away, but my words shall not pass away."

Another spiritual figure who lived thousands of years ago and who also possessed and spoke with divine authority was the avatar Rama of India. The healing potencies of some Rama mantras are among the most powerful I have ever encountered. The following story about Rama tells us much with regard to healing ourselves.

The Spiritual Power of Rama.
Rama was heir to the royal throne in the kingdom where he grew up. But through a series of incidents arising from court intrigue, he was forced to spend twelve years in exile in the forest. His exile was part of a divine design. In those years, he was able to bless many people who might not otherwise have met him.

While traveling with Lakshmana, his brother, he came upon a slab of rock and purposefully trod upon it. The rock immediately assumed the form of a woman, who bowed down before him. The woman thanked him and he blessed her and moved on. A hundred years earlier she had been cursed by a sage in a moment of anger. So powerful were his words that she remained in a rocklike state until Rama, with his divine authority, arrived.

The news of Rama's deed spread quickly, as such matters do. Two days later, Rama arrived at a broad river that could be crossed only by ferry. The local ferry was a small rowboat operated by a man named Guha.

In those days it was considered a great blessing to touch the feet of a holy person. The reason for this is that there are very large chakras in the feet. In most of us these chakras remain closed, because the current that would flow from them is too strong for us until we have evolved to a certain spiritual level.

In the New Testament, we find Jesus washing the feet of the disciples. Even when they object, Jesus tells them that he must do this for them: "What I do now you do not understand, but you will later when I send the Holy Spirit." Jesus is providing one of the last steps of spiritual initiation for his disciples. He is opening the chakras in their feet. After Baptism with the Holy Spirit, their feet chakras will blaze with a powerful spiritual energy. At that point, great spiritual energy pours forth from the activated chakras in the feet.

The tradition of honoring the feet of the spiritually advanced has continued in the Far East for thousands of years. Even today, traditional Hindus and Buddhists will bow down to touch the feet of ones they revere—in some cases receiving a jolt of an electrical type of energy.

Now Guha had heard of the great event in which Rama's treading upon the rock had caused a woman to materialize. He had been filled with joy, but also troubled because he knew Rama's path would take him across the river for which Guha himself was the only boatman. Guha waited in seeming quiet as Rama approached his boat. Inside, Guha's thoughts were racing. What might happen to his boat if Rama came aboard? Might the boat turn into a woman? Or some object other than a boat? As he considered several possibilities, he arrived at the best solution he could come up with.

Rama and Lakshmana greeted Guha pleasantly and asked to be taken across to the other side. Guha replied, "Oh Rama, I have heard that the dust from your feet turned a rock into a woman. I have no other means of subsistence for my family than this small boat. If you would ride with me, please allow me to wash your feet so that the dust will not turn my boat into someone else."

Rama was very pleased to hear the artful yet devoted words of Guha. He consented to have his feet washed by Guha, who became bathed in the tremendous spiritual energy springing from them endlessly, peacefully, and powerfully. With tears of devotion streaming down his cheeks, Guha applied water and gentle soap to the glowing feet.

When he had finished, Rama and Lakshmana entered into the boat and Guha ferried them to the opposite shore. Then Rama asked Guha what his charges were. Guha replied, "By your grace I have taken you across a river. You kindly take me across the ocean of this samsara." Samsara is the ocean of rebirth. Guha wanted to be liberated from the necessity of being reborn again and again until he achieved liberation from the continuing cycle of rebirth.

Rama, very much pleased at the words of Guha, replied, "Your devotion is such as I have rarely seen. It shall be as you request. Henceforth you will be reborn only by your own choice. Also, because of your devotion, ask a favor and I will grant it."

Guha thought for a moment and said, "It is my desire that the very name of Rama be superior to all other mantras in the removal of the sins one may have accumulated."

Rama smiled and replied, "So be it," and departed from the river.

From this story has developed a stockpile of Rama mantras that work very powerfully in digging up and neutralizing negative karma.

A Simple and Powerful Healing Rama Mantra.

Om Ram Ramaya Namaha

(OM RAHM RAHM-EYE-YAH NAHM-AH-HA)

Ram has a twofold meaning and application in Sanskrit. First, it is the seed sound for the manipura, or solar plexus chakra. Tremendous healing energy lies dormant at that chakra. Mantra can help you get at the energy. This mantra begins to awaken and activate the entire chakra. It specifically prepares the chakra to be able to handle the inflow of kundalini energy that gives the chakra its power.

The second application involves dividing *Rama* into the syllables *Ra* and *Ma*. *Ra* is associated with the solar current that runs down the right side of our bodies. *Ma* is associated with the lunar current that runs down the left side of our bodies. Although these two currents crisscross and meet at the chakras, they are generally associated with the right and left sides of the body. By repeating *Rama . . . Rama . . . Rama* over and over again, you begin balancing the two currents and their activity so that they can work with the higher stages of energy that will eventually come up the spine. This simple mantra, *Rama*, qualifies as a healing mantra in its own right.

The simple mantra *Om Ram Ramaya Namaha* begins to clear the two currents with a slight emphasis on the right or solar side, which is needed in this age of darkness. As discussed in chapter 6, after the age of twenty-nine, the ending of the mantra should be changed to *Swaha*. At the Saturn Return around the age of twenty-nine, the energy pattern in the body changes. Our general energy center rises from the second chakra to the third chakra.

Long and Powerful Rama Healing Mantra.
Of all the mantras I have ever used for healing purposes, I consider this one of the most powerful. I am aware that it is long, but I teach it even to beginners because of the tremendous healing power it produces. I have found that those who are desperate for healing learn it without difficulty, and many have had extraordinary results. This is one of the mantras Cynthia used to recover from her twenty-year bout with fibromyalgia. At the time she undertook the mantra discipline, she had barely even heard of mantras. Yet even as a beginner she was able to achieve dramatic and powerful results. Here is the long Rama healing mantra, with a very rough translation:

Om Apa-damapa Hataram Dataram Sarva Sampadam Loka Bhi Ramam Sri Ramam Bhuyo Bhuyo Namam-yaham

(OM AP-PAH-DAH-MAH-PAH HAH-TAH-RAHM DAH-TAH-RAHM
SAHR-VAH SAHM-PAH-DAHM LOH-KAH BEE RAHM-AHM SHREE
RAHM-MAHM BOO-YOH BOO-YOH NAH-MAHM-YAH-HAHM)

"Om. O most compassionate Rama. Please send your
healing energy right here to the Earth, to the Earth
[twice for emphasis]. Salutations."

Although the mantra is long, it is simple to say phonetically. If you can, say it 108 times in a sitting. If you are just starting out, this may initially take up to one hour. After you are comfortable with the mantra, it will only take you thirty minutes. If you are very familiar with the mantra, 108 repetitions can be accomplished in twenty minutes.

Rama Mantra as Pain Medication.
Judy suffered constant pain for four years. She undertook a discipline with this mantra, and after just a few weeks, her pain decreased to less pain than at any time she could remember. She is still doing the mantra and expects to be pain-free relatively soon.

Mantras for
Mental Health and Reunion

A woman that my wife and I know has a son on medication for bipolar disorder. Recently, spurning his pills, he had taken off from home and disappeared for a time. His family, not knowing where he was or how he was faring, worried greatly. The woman decided to do a forty-day discipline with the long Rama healing mantra. After she had completed the discipline on his behalf, he soon returned home, went back on his medication, and stabilized his life. Another couple I know chanted this mantra for forty days and were led to a physician who helped their mentally ill son find a beneficial new course of treatment.

Please be aware that mantra meditation is not intended as a replacement for other therapies. In the cases we've just discussed, medical and holistic healing methods were still being used, but the patients or their families said their mantras and watched for guidance. There is a common human temptation to hope for a miraculous solution to our difficulties, instead of working toward a solution. As you use a healing mantra, stay open to receiving information and unexpected aid.

A Nervous Condition

Hector had a most unusual problem. From the age of ten, he would sweat profusely from his hands. He could not shake hands with anyone without being terribly embarrassed by clammy palms. Doctor after doctor told him that his was a rare condition about which they could do nothing. Hector soon became shy and withdrawn. One day when he was in his late teens he saw an article describing how a Swiss medical clinic had devised a treatment for just such a problem. The procedure involved going into the nerves along the spine that control sweating of the hands, and tying them off so that the automatic sweating simply disappeared.

It took several months of judicious saving before Hector could afford the $10,000 price and the airfare. He even gave up his living quarters and slept outside for a short time to save money. Finally he had enough funds and he made arrangements with the clinic and traveled to Switzerland for the operation.

It worked. For about a month. Now he experienced a new problem. While his hands were just fine, he started sweating profusely from his abdomen. It got so bad he could not wear light colors; only dark sport shirts and sweatshirts made their way into his closet.

Hector told this story in a class on mantra I was teaching, some two months after the course had begun. His fellow students and I couldn't help but notice that he was wearing a light-colored sportshirt and it was completely dry. He said that after hearing about the long Rama healing mantra, he became inspired to give it a try. Hector told us he was not temperamentally suited to sitting formally for meditation, so he just said the mantra as often as he could all day long. He said it going to sleep, waking up, and off and on during the day. After just three weeks, his sweating problem began to subside. He continued the mantra for two more weeks and the problem went away completely.

Hector shed some tears as he told this story, but then he grinned as he touched his completely dry, cream-colored shirt. He still says the mantra because he likes the way it makes him feel.

Markandeya Mantra for Viral Infection

Connie already knew that she was sick when she kept her second appointment with the doctor. Diagnosed with bronchial pneumonia, she thought the antibiotic was not doing the job after she had taken it for three weeks. She was right. A rare virus that had invaded her system was causing her to lose cartilage all over her body. She did not respond to treatment for that condition. With an ashen face, the doctor told her she probably had about six months to live.

Diving into the world of alternative therapies and treatments, Connie was determined to beat the virus. After six months of trying various cures with some encouraging results, she decided to apply yet another offbeat therapy: Sanskrit mantra. She chose the Markandeya mantra, or Maha-Mrityunjaya mantra, which was mentioned in chapter 3. It is considered one of the most potent healing mantras in the world.

Here is the classical story surrounding Markandeya and the great healing mantra for which he is the seer.

The sage Mrikandu and his wife led saintly lives, performing the divine meditations and rituals with humility and devotion. Although they had achieved great spiritual knowledge, strength, and wisdom, they had no children. In a meditation they performed with the intention of fulfilling this desire, they experienced a visitation from Lord Shiva himself, who offered them the choice of a divine son who would live only sixteen years, or a bad son who would live one hundred years. Shiva knew well their choice in advance and was not surprised when they chose the divine child. Their desires from long ago were fulfilled and they had a divine son whom they named Markandeya.

This advanced spiritual couple had much to impart to their son, including the Gayatri mantra and Shiva puja, which he performed every day with great devotion. Over his first fifteen years they gave him the tools to attain spiritual knowledge. They never told him about the shortness of his life span.

On his sixteenth birthday, Markandeya finished his Gayatri mantra meditation and began his puja as usual. Halfway through the ceremony, he felt his prana start to leave his body and immediately knew he was dying. Stricken with fear and grief, he thought of Shiva, thought of his parents, and threw his arms around the Shiva-lingam, the symbol of the Shiva's energy and form. He uttered the following prayer:

Om Trayumbakam Yajamahe Sughandhim Pushti Vardanam Urvar-ukamiva Bandhanan Mrityor Muksheeya Mamritat

(OM TRY-UM-BAH-KUM YA-JAHM-MAH-HEY SOO-GAHN-DIM
POOSH-TEE VAHR-DAH-NAHM OOR-VAHR-OO-KUMEE-VAH BAHN-
DAHN-AHN MRIT-YOUR MOOK-SHEE-YAH MAHM-REE-TAHT)

*"Shelter me, O three-eyed Lord Shiva. Bless me with health
and immortality and sever me from the clutches of death,
even as a cucumber is cut from its creeper."*

Shiva appeared to the boy and made this pronouncement: "It is true that your karma decrees that you must die at the age of sixteen. However, you have not yet quite reached your sixteenth birthday. It is still a few minutes away. Therefore, I stop your aging process at this very moment. You shall not get any older. Thus, death may never claim you." So saying, Shiva disappeared. Even to this day in classical Hindu studies, Markandeya is referred to as one of the ever-living masters whose abode is high up in the Himalayas.

Around this story, in India, has arisen a powerful spiritual discipline that is used to promote healing. Although priests perform pujas and fire ceremonies for others using this mantra, the classical form of the mantra discipline is meant to be performed by the person himself or herself. Called the Maha-Mrityunjaya mantra, which roughly means "great mantra relieving one from death and disease," this mantra is often referred to in everyday discussions as the Markandeya mantra. It is efficacious for relief of a wide variety of chronic illnesses, including immune system problems. Of course, it is no substitute for conventional medical care.

Connie repeated this mantra 108 times morning and evening for three months. She got much better. Twelve months later she still said her Markandeya mantra every day while continuing to improve. After working with the mantra for four months, she even went horseback riding. Currently she is living an active and healthy life. She recently got married, and the virus has almost disappeared as of this writing, over a year after she was given six months to live.

Intuition Can Guide You to Your Mantra

To try to find the right mantra for a specific condition not covered here, briefly try out each of the mantras presented in this chapter. After a few repetitions, one or two of them may seem to resonate with you more than others. You may be drawn to the Dhanvantre mantra, or one of the Rama mantras, or the Markandeya mantra. Try out one for a longer period—a day or two—to see if your body and mind respond.

Once you have selected a mantra, be disciplined and diligent. Keep open to healing messages or opportunities that present themselves. If it appears that nothing is happening, another more powerful force may be at work in your life, one that you may not yet comprehend. It may be that an agreement your soul made before occupying this body is obstructing the result you seek.

Similarly, if you are chanting for someone else, you may find that your efforts do not produce the result you desire. Sometimes a person's

karma is so entrenched that healing cannot take place, or that person
has a karmic task to live with serious illness. Sometimes illness claims
our loved ones because their time in this incarnation has been fulfilled.

Karma Rules

I once performed a healing discipline on behalf of a family member
who had cancer. It was the longest and strongest discipline I have ever
done for another person. I said the long, healing rama mantras every
day for 120 days. My wife worked with this mantra for this healing
even harder than I did. After 40 days, 80 days, and 115 days we performed a healing fire ceremony that I knew from experience to be extremely powerful. I had seen so many near-miraculous things over the
years that resulted from mantra disciplines that I was confident my
relative would get well. I was wrong.

I had contracted with myself and with her to do a 120-day discipline. She also did her part daily, chanting a shorter mantra. She died
on EXACTLY the one-hundred-twentieth day of my discipline. I had
literally just finished my meditation at seven in the morning when the
phone rang. It was her husband, calling to tell me that she had passed
away. I was thunderstruck.

A few days later, after I had recovered from my shock, I sat down
and went into deep meditation. My object was to discern what had
gone wrong. I was so certain she would live. Had I erred someplace?
Was my discipline faulty? After some time, images and thoughts began
to form in my mind in a most amazing way, and I believed they were
messages about this relative's life purpose and path. I saw that she had
never intended to stay very long in the body from which she had just
disengaged, and that she would be reborn to a wonderful spiritual
family with almost an ideal life. Many things she might have wanted
for this life, but which had not happened, would be fulfilled in her
next life. Her acceptance of mantra as a spiritual discipline—she knew
nothing about Sanskrit mantra until she got cancer—would pay off
handsomely in her very next life. All of the efforts made on her behalf

would also manifest for her in the next life. As the ancient saying goes, "Put forth your efforts and leave the rest to God."

Spiritual energy obeys laws just as physical energy does, and we all know that the energy is never lost. So rest assured that your efforts are never wasted. By your mantra discipline, whether for yourself or someone else, you have set forces into motion that will produce a positive result somewhere along the line. In matters of health, I have learned to append to all my healing prayers the ending, "Nevertheless, not my will but Thy will, O Lord."

8

Mantras for Mastering Fear

As we might expect from the author of *Alice's Adventures in Wonderland*, Charles Dodgson (Lewis Carroll) was an insightful if eccentric philosopher. Dodgson believed that happiness exists only in the past: we remember happiness rather than know it in the moment. Knowing it, after all, would introduce an element of intellectual distance that is inimical to genuine happiness. Self-consciousness subverts spontaneity, in other words, and spontaneity is fundamental to having a really good time.

But if happiness can exist only in the past, perhaps fear can exist only in the present. Just think of a few things that really frightened you at various points in your life. Were you afraid of bugs? Of ghosts? Of the deep end of the swimming pool? Of not getting a date for the prom? Although you may be able to remember how those fears felt, chances are you don't experience them now with anything like their original power. Moreover, the things you're afraid of today will probably seem just as harmless when you look back at them over a distance of years—which doesn't mean that they aren't very frightening now.

Dealing effectively with fear does not mean just getting rid of it. There are people who break the law and who aren't afraid to die in the process, but that's not a state of mind we should aspire to. A hungry jackass will keep eating until he makes himself sick, heedless of wolves, a hailstorm, or a sharp blow with a stick. The jackass has overcome his fear, but that's only a negative accomplishment. He may not be frightened, but he's not effective at living, either.

We might not be able to define them precisely, but we intuitively recognize the differences between rash acts and the things that become possible when fear is extinguished and is replaced by courage, hope, or love. Fear doesn't even need to be replaced. It is our fear of fear that is misplaced. Aristotle may have had this in mind when he wrote, "A truly courageous person is not someone who never feels fear, but someone who fears the right thing, at the right time, in the right way."

NASA has documented that its astronauts were not frightened at all under some extremely hazardous conditions. They fit Aristotle's view perfectly. As explorers who knew they were risking much, the astronauts, when confronted with sudden dangerous, unpredicted problems, did not exhibit fear as most of us would have under similar conditions. They simply took the most effective action available to them and watched carefully for other opportunities to address problems and dangers. The important lesson here is that there are times when an attitude driven by fear is not helpful, but just gets in the way.

Conversely, the energy of fear can also be a useful thing. For some actors, stage fright is useful. Most stage fright occurs before the actor walks onstage. Once on, the energy of stage fright propels the performance.

This chapter, therefore, will not show you how to use mantras simply to banish fear. Instead, it will provide mantras for dealing well with fear, for protection within the consciousness from the feared object or state, and even for using fear to achieve worthwhile purposes. Fear is a powerful form of energy, and anything that strong shouldn't be discarded carelessly, but transformed if possible.

Tolstoy wrote that all fears, even trivial ones, really are fears of death. But death is a word, not a thought. Fear of death is really fear of helplessness. The common fear of death is the fear of losing all power.

The Eastern teachings about death are quite different from Western views. In the West, death is considered a finality; in the East, death is just another door the soul enters when time in that body comes to an end. Soon there will be another birth and another body. It is not surprising, then, that in classical religious households in the East, death may be dreaded but is not feared. The dread is of the inevitable march toward a time and place in the unknown, but the fear of the finality of death is not an issue.

The fear of helplessness manifests as inaction and paralysis—physical, emotional, and spiritual—which are much more dangerous than the fear itself. That's the fear of a deer frozen in the headlights of a car, waiting for the impact, and by waiting making the impact inevitable. People who master fear strive to make the most of every moment today. What they do fear is not finding and fulfilling the purpose that brought them to this lifetime. They fear the impulse to dominate other people, or be dominated by them. They fear making appearances more important than realities. They fear seeing themselves as more important than those who depend on them. Most important, they use those fears as a source of energy for their personal spiritual evolution and transformation. That's the ultimate purpose of the general mantras to combat and transform fear.

A saying from the East is, "Fear is the beginning of knowledge." You may sense danger before you consciously apprehend it. A heightened nervousness or portentousness signals the conscious mind that something is not right, that some threat is brewing or imminent.

Clinical studies at the University of Michigan, conducted by R. B. Zajonc in 1979, strongly support the conclusion that there are two independent systems of knowledge operating in the human body/consciousness. One is based upon cognition and the other upon affect. The research found that these two systems of knowledge do not both operate at the same time or under all conditions. The findings explain why we can have this eerie feeling that something is wrong when there is nothing tangible we can point to. The system of knowledge based upon affect is telling the body that something is not right. The conscious mind picks up this conclusion and begins to cognize or think about it. The sensory apparatus comes under heightened attention as we survey our situation, trying to recognize consciously what the feeling system has been telling us. In the West, we sometimes call this phenomenon intuition.

The intuitive system of knowledge is no more perfect than the one based upon cognition. Just as we can analyze a situation and come to completely false conclusions, so, too, can we experience a fear or anxiety that turns out to have no basis in reality at all. So, to deal with the phenomenon of fear, we must rely upon a philosophic approach common to allopathic medicine: we must treat the symptoms.

The first antidote to fear presented is a mantra that invokes protection. Subsequent mantras provide remedies for specific kinds of fear. Finally, we'll work on transforming the energy of fear. Like the mantras presented in the chapter on healing, most mantras for dealing with fear are general in nature. A general mantra can, however, work for specific circumstances if your intention is clear. The following incident illustrates this point.

Protection When You Need It

Like most college students, Rick liked rock and roll. When one of his favorite bands was scheduled to appear at the local arena, he and a buddy got good tickets three months in advance. Then Rick enrolled in one of my courses on mantras for dealing with life's problems. Drawn immediately to the Eastern feminine trinity of Durga, Lakshmi, and Saraswati, Rick decided to complete a classical forty-day discipline dedicated to each one. He wanted to awaken those powerful feminine qualities within himself: Lakshmi for abundance, Durga for protection, and Saraswati for knowledge.

Durga is portrayed in India as the divine protectress. Riding astride a lion or tiger, she is beautiful to behold yet has a hundred arms, each with a different weapon. The lore describes her as beautiful to the devotee of truth and terrible to the demonic force that attempts to harm good people who place their trust in her.

Rick was halfway through his forty-day mantra discipline on Durga when the date for the concert arrived. As he and his friend pulled into the parking lot, Rick knew everything was not right. He could feel increasing tension in his solar plexus. The farther into the lot they drove, the more it increased, until he began to feel sick to his stomach. He remembered his Durga mantra for protection and began to chant it silently, without any idea of what lay ahead.

Om Dum Durgayei Namaha

(OM DOOM DOOR-GAH-YEI NAHM-AH-HA)

He continuously said the mantra silently as they slid into a parking place. Also feeling nervous, Rick's friend asked him to lead them both on the long journey from the fringes of the parking lot to the arena entrance. Rick assented and, chanting in a mumbling tone, led them on a zigzag route. Sensing trouble from time to time, he narrowly avoided a drunken brawl already brewing down one parking aisle. Quickly changing lanes, he saw a woman lying on the ground holding her stomach. Even though he wanted to keep going, something inside would not let him. As he stopped and knelt down, she told him she was feeling sick and wanted to leave but was too overcome by nausea. Instinctively he grabbed her hand and began to chant the Durga mantra. Within a few minutes she felt better and was able to get in her car and leave the parking lot.

Weaving from row to row and still chanting, Rick and his friend made their way toward the entrance. At one point Rick saw police rousting people from a tailgate party and at another he warned a group smoking something illegal that the cops were on the prowl. Within another few minutes they were inside the arena and in their seats. Later, I asked Rick if he had liked the concert. "It was great," he said. "But I guess Durga was protecting all kinds of people." I could hardly disagree.

This mantra is easy to say and memorize. Let the power of the anthropomorphized feminine energy of protection, Durga, be handy in your spiritual toolbox, readily available in your time of need, just as it was for Rick.

The following is a more specific mantra for fear.

Mantra to Remove Ghosts or the Fear of Unwanted Spirits

Shiva is a personification of consciousness in its expanded and most powerful state of being and accomplishment. In the teachings of the East, this consciousness extends from the nether spheres inhabited by ghosts, disembodied spirits, goblins, and demons to the highest celestial realms where the sages and saints dwell. This mantra commands that spirits or beings who are not in their proper place return to their correct plane of consciousness.

Om Apa-sarpantu Tae Bhuta Yei Bhuta
Bhuvi Sam-stitaha
Yei Bhuta Vigna Kartara
Stei Gachantu Shiva Ajnaya

(OM AH-PA-SAHR-PAHN-TOO TEH BOOTA YEA BOOTA

BOO-VEE SAHM-STEE-TAH-HA

YEA BOOTAH VIG-NAH KAHR-TAH-RAH

STEA GAH-CHAHN-TOO SHEE-VAH AHJ-NAH-YAH)

"May the spirits that are haunting this area leave and never return, by the order of Shiva."

The Pillar of Light

An ancient fable showing the infinite extension of consciousness goes like this: Brahma and Vishnu were traveling in the vast expanses of the universe one day when they came upon a pillar of light. It extended both upward and downward until it was lost from view. Curious about it, they agreed they would each travel in one of its directions, find the starting point, and return to compare notes. So deciding, they took off in rapid flight characteristic of the advanced state of their being. After several eons of flight with no end to the pillar of light coming into view, Vishnu returned to the place where he and Brahma had first discovered it. Shortly after his return, Brahma similarly returned to their starting place. Vishnu spoke first, saying, "I was unable to find its beginning." Lying, Brahma responded that he had found an end to the pillar. Immediately upon Brahma's statement, the pillar turned into Shiva, who spoke to them. "Brahma has lied. I, Shiva, am the pillar of light and consciousness which has no beginning and no end."

Because he lied, Brahma was made to suffer neglect during observance of the divine ceremonies. In India today, there are very few pujas or observances to Brahma. It is understood that the lesson in this for humanity is that when we become powerful, ego often asserts itself in negative ways. Vishnu's work of constantly teaching and helping the evolution of consciousness has automatically kept his ego in check through service to others.

In esoteric learning circles, the pillar of light is taught as the human spine: the seat of consciousness and the road of evolution combined. Shiva is that state of consciousness which is our essential nature, with dominion over all substates of consciousness as represented by individual beings, either real or imagined. So when a negative force is told to leave the area by order of Shiva, through the medium of mantra as described in reference to the previous Shiva mantra, the effect is powerful.

Mantra to Remove Fear of Loneliness and Provide Companionship

If you have a friendly nature, you will never be without friends or companions. This mantra helps develop the energy of friendship within you.

═══════════════════════════════════════

Om Hraum Mitraya Namaha

(OM HROUWM MEE-TRAH-YAH NAHM-AH-HA)

*"May the light of friendship shine through me,
drawing noble companionship."*

═══════════════════════════════════════

Mantra to Transform the Energy of Fear

Another approach to removing fear is to transform it. When fear is dissolved back to its original source in consciousness, its energy is released, and becomes available to be used in creative and productive ways.

═══════════════════════════════════════

Shante Prashante Sarva Bhaya Upasha Mani Swaha

(SHAN-TEH PRAH-SHAN-TEH SAHR-VAH BHAH-YAH

OO-PAH-SHAH MAH-NEE SWAH-HA)

*"Invoking supreme peace I offer [surrender] the quality of fear to its
source in the higher and formless universal mind. Salutations."*

═══════════════════════════════════════

This approach to transforming fear is based upon the idea of dispersion. It assumes that fear is a concentration of energy in an undesirable form. Once that concentration of energy is dissipated, a state of genuine serenity becomes possible—the state known in Sanskrit as *shanti*.

9

Mantras for Anger and Other Undesirable Inner Conditions

We all have characteristics that we wish we could change. Inner states such as despair, grief, jealousy, and anger can be disruptive and destructive to our outer lives. Anger can permanently alienate other people. An angry person may have difficulty in getting and holding a job. A jealous person may find that relationships are short-lived and unpleasant, however much intentions run to the opposite. A prideful or arrogant person may end up alone because he or she acts "so much better than anyone else."

The outer results from these and other inner conditions may be similar, but the causes are somewhat different. In Sanskrit mantra, these inner conditions all have names that relate to the vibration of the state they represent. For anger, the Sanskrit word is *krodha*. Even if you have never heard the word before, you may experience a certain constriction in the subtle body upon reading it. That constriction is unpleasant and counterproductive to a peaceful and successful outer life. If you know the inner condition that is causing a problem, there is an excellent chance that mantras can help you deal with it.

Although there are times when it may be difficult to get a clear picture of what your particular inner condition is, a good friend, spouse, minister, or psychotherapist can help you. If you have had a loved one die recently, grief and anger can easily be identified as causing difficulties. If a relationship is characterized by constant fighting, there may be more than one cause. For instance, one party may be overly controlling while the other suffers from indecision. While diagnosing these inner conditions is difficult, it becomes easier if you or the person with the problem genuinely wants relief.

Where relief is genuinely sought, Sanskrit mantra formulas can be extremely useful. Recognizing these inner conditions millennia ago, sages and seers have passed down Sanskrit mantras that can help reduce and eventually eliminate anger as well as other undesirable inner conditions. The basic formula used to reduce or eliminate anger also lends itself to elimination of other conditions that may stand in your way, as will be shown a little later.

Habitual and Chronic

Before going into those formulas, we would do well to remember that these inner states qualify as chronic conditions. If we struggle with anger, it is not that one day we suddenly begin to manifest anger. Usually it established a foothold early in our life, and then became part of our personality. So two things are important to note: First, at some level, anger has become a habit. Second, habits seem to "defend themselves."

People who have tried to stop smoking will tell you of the problems involved: of breaking down and sneaking a cigarette, or recommitting to stopping again but repeatedly falling off the wagon. The reason is that the habit has established its own energy center within. The smoker, in breaking the habit, is really trying to reclaim misappropriated energy that has become crystallized in a negative way. A useful insight lies in this catchphrase from psychology: "Find your anger and there you will find your energy."

The Sanskrit approach to changing the undesirable inner conditions is directly tied to changing the energy pattern. The vibration of the mantra goes immediately to the negative condition and begins to break it up. As a result, there may be some outer "drama" that takes place somewhere in the process as the energy center "defends itself." We may get very angry over something trivial. Such a reaction can be mild or strong, depending upon the particulars of the person and the depth of the problem.

To change a chronic condition, there are three phases for which mantra practice is employed. Using medical treatment as a model, we can describe the process like this:

- Vibratory intervention or surgery, which takes place over a period of days or weeks as the condition is transformed;
- A dressing or unguent, which begins to rearrange the energy into a new and useful pattern;
- A bandage, which slowly turns to new skin protecting the place where the transformation took place.

Surgical Intervention

The basic mantra for transforming one of these inner conditions is:

Shante Prashante Sarva ——— Upasha Mani Swaha

(SHAN-TEH PRA-SHAN-TEH SAHR-VAH ——— OO-PASH-AH

MAH-NEE SWA-HA)

The first two words relate to the Sanskrit word for peace, *shanti*. *Sarva* denotes the source of the condition we are addressing, and which is to be offered or given up. *Upasha Mani* means surrendering the smaller aspect of mind to the universal "mind without form." *Swaha* means "I offer with salutations." Thus, the surface meaning of the mantra is: "Invoking supreme peace I offer (surrender) the quality of _____ to its source in the higher and formless universal mind. Salutations."

The Sanskrit word for anger, as mentioned earlier, is *krodha*. The mantra for elimination of anger is, therefore:

Shante Prashante Sarva Krodha Upasha Mani Swaha

(SHAN-TEH PRA-SHAN-TEH SAHR-VAH KROH-DHA

OO-PASH-AH MAH-NEE SWA-HA)

In 1977 I undertook a forty-day discipline of this mantra to attack an inner condition of irritability. I was living in conditions that were very stressful, with little chance to relax and re-center. Although there may have been a good explanation for my state, there was still no excuse for my shortness with others. I simply did not like my own behavior during this period and decided that there were much better ways of reacting and behaving, even within the confines of an unpleasant situation.

After forty days of mantra practice, the condition of irritability had subsided greatly. I even made peace with someone with whom I had been quarreling for some time. After the initial truce, we discovered that we had many things in common and became very good friends. One of the lessons in all this for me was that, due to my inner condition, I had been unable to see a potential good friend, even when I saw that person every day. Any of these inner conditions can temporarily blind you to good things right in front of you.

Adding Salve

Although the discipline was successful, I felt somewhat raw at the conclusion of it. Over the intervening years, I have discovered mantras that could have placed a balm on that rawness. Now that I have accumulated more mantras and better understanding, I can help smooth your work to change negative inner conditions.

Here is a mantra for easing a recently transformed negative energy pattern into a positive one. It will ease the transition of your energy to a new and pleasant state. You may practice this mantra for forty days after the "surgical intervention" mantra. A little later I will present a complete sixty-day practice using three mantras, including this one.

Om Sri Maha Lakshmiyei Swaha

(OM SHREE MAH-HA LAKSH-MEE-YEI SWAH-HA)

"Om and salutations. I invoke the Great Feminine Principle of Great Abundance."

The energy of abundance is *Lakshmi* in Sanskrit. *Maha* can mean "great" in one application, and it is related to the heart center in another context. Here, both applications are appropriate.

Abundance is usually thought of as simple prosperity, but it is far more. *Any form of abundance* is the core meaning. Thus it can be friends as wealth, enough food as wealth, good health as wealth, good family relations as wealth, and so on. The highest state of abundance is love. It is the pinnacle of every good and abundant thing.

The mantra for great abundance can be used as a salve. It becomes an unguent to soothe the newly disrupted energy pattern, which, although now transformed, has left a raw place in the personality. The personality must adjust to the lack of a previous way of behaving. The mind and personality must catch up to the changes in energy. This mantra will aid greatly in the peaceful and harmonious transition to new and positive energy states.

Bandaging and
Building New Skin

The process of converting an old energy pattern to a new one now needs a final, "bandage" mantra. This mantra is simple and can be practiced for a full forty days after completing the "surgical intervention" mantra and the Lakshmi mantra of great abundance, or it can be included in the twenty-plus-twenty-plus-twenty-day practice I will explain shortly.

Om Shanti Om

(OM SHAHN-TEE OM)

"Om, Dynamic Peace, Om."

Om is the seed sound for the brow center, which is where the masculine and feminine energies meet. *Shanti* means peace in a dynamic sense: not just an empty shell, but a powerful and active peace that radiates outward. This mantra gives the personality an entirely new energy to work with, in tandem with the Lakshmi energy. At the energy level, the combination of these two mantras completely replaces the crystallized anger center with a new and positive vibration. Transformation of the previous condition is now complete.

Methods for Practice

As explained in chapter 3, the traditional approach to mantra discipline falls into one of two categories: the forty-day discipline, or the goal of a certain number of repetitions. For optimum results in transforming a lifelong pattern, the first mantra should be chanted as frequently as possible for forty days in succession, then the next one for another forty days, and the final one for another forty. This would produce a total discipline of 120 days.

A shorter, more incremental approach can also work. Instead of chanting each mantra as much as possible for forty days, chant each one for twenty days and then move on to the next. The total program will take sixty days. Then stop. Watch what happens. I call this the 20-20-20 approach.

Do not undertake another discipline like this for at least two weeks. This will allow you some distance to assess your progress. It will also give your mind and personality a break. They have been working hard. Now give them a rest. After two weeks, if you see progress that inspires you and you would like to work further with this or another condition, then start again.

The Very Gentle Approach

If you would like to stick your toe in the water before you dive in, another way you can begin to experiment with mantras for changing negative chronic and habitual inner conditions is by setting aside a time twice a day for your practice. Use the 20-20-20 approach, but instead of saying the mantra as much as possible, say it 108 times in the morning and 108 times in the evening. For the first twenty days, work with the first mantra twice a day instead of all day long during your normal activities. For the second twenty days, work with the "salve" or "unguent" mantra the same way: twice a day for 108 times. The third 20 days, do the same with the Shanti mantra. This sixty-day discipline will give you a good taste of the mantras and how they work. Results will vary from person to person.

Other Inner Conditions

So far we have addressed only anger as an inner condition to be changed. Many others are listed below in English and Sanskrit. The specific "first" mantra for each energy state is shown. This list applies only to your work during the first part of the program. The other two parts remain exactly the same, using the Lakshmi mantra and the Shanti mantra.

Mantras for
Specific Inner Conditions

Anger (general condition)	*Krodha*	*Shante Prashante Sarva Krodha Upasha Mani Swaha*
Anger (between two people)	*Mah-na*	*Shante Prashante Sarva Mah-Na Upasha Mani Swaha*
Pride	*Mada*	*Shante Prashante Sarva Mada Upasha Mani Swaha*
Envy	*Matsarya*	*Shante Prashante Sarva Matsarya Upasha Mani Swaha*
Ignorance/Delusion	*Moha*	*Shante Prashante Sarva Moha Upasha Mani Swaha*
Covetousness	*Lobha*	*Shante Prashante Sarva Lobha Upasha Mani Swaha*
Consuming lust	*Kama*	*Shante Prashante Sarva Kama Upasha Mani Swaha*
Mistrust/Suspiciousness	*Avish-Vasa*	*Shante Prashante Sarva Avish-Vasa Upasha Mani Swaha*
Shame	*Laja*	*Shante Prashante Sarva Laja Upasha Mani Swaha*
Fickleness	*Pishu-Nata*	*Shante Prashante Sarva Pishu-Nata Upasha Mani Swaha*
Fear	*Bhaya*	*Shante Prashante Sarva Bhaya Upasha Mani Swaha*
Jealousy	*Irsha*	*Shante Prashante Sarva Irsha Upasha Mani Swaha*
Aversion/Disgust	*Ghrina*	*Shante Prashante Sarva Ghrina Upasha Mani Swaha*
Arrogance	*Dambha*	*Shante Prashante Sarva Dambha Upasha Mani Swaha*
Conceit	*Ahankara*	*Shante Prashante Sarva Ahankara Upasha Mani Swaha*
Grief	*Shoka*	*Shante Prashante Sarva Shoka Upasha Mani Swaha*

Dejection	*Kheda*	*Shante Prashante Sarva Kheda Upasha Mani Swaha*
Agitation	*Sam-Bhrama*	*Shante Prashante Sarva Sam-Bhrama Upasha Mani Swaha*
Laziness	*Shu-Shupti*	*Shante Prashante Sarva Shu-Shupti Upasha Mani Swaha*
Sadness	*Vishada*	*Shante Prashante Sarva Vishada Upasha Mani Swaha*
Duplicity	*Kapata-Ta*	*Shante Prashante Sarva Kapata-Ta Upasha Mani Swaha*

These mantra formulas and the 60-day or 120-day programs should never be forced upon anyone. You should not even attempt to be persuasive about their use. If you feel drawn to use the mantra formulas, then by all means begin your discipline. If you find that you are thinking of someone who would benefit from this approach to changing inner conditions, then by all means recommend these methods. But remember, you are working with karma. That means that nothing should be forced. As they say in the East, "You cannot rip the skin from the snake. It must shed it by itself."

Mantra for Reducing Fear and Anger, and for Spiritual Liberation

Here is another mantra for transforming anger and fear. This great mantra was practiced by Mahatma Gandhi from the time he was a young boy.

Om Sri Rama Jaya Rama, Jaya Jaya Rama

(OM SHREE RAH-MAH JAH-YAH RAH-MAH,
JAH-YAH JAH-YAH RAH-MAH)

*"Om to Rama and his consort [represented by Sri]
victory to Rama, victory, victory again to Rama."*

This is called the Taraka mantra, which means "that which takes one across" the ocean of rebirth. The component sounds of the mantra are as follows:

Om is the mantra seed sound for the brow center located between the eyebrows and three-quarters of an inch above. *Sri* is a mantra that both salutes and activates the feminine power located at the base of the spine. *Rama* refers to the seventh avatar of Vishnu in one context, and to the divine self located in all of us in another context. *Jaya* means victory.

Since liberation from continued rebirth is a foundation goal of the Hindu religion, the Taraka mantra is commonly practiced by orthodox Hindus for this purpose.

Mahatma Gandhi learned it from his nurse while still a young boy. No famous spiritual teacher gave him this mantra. The simple yet powerful faith of his nurse imbued the mantra with power.

Through his devotion to truth and nonviolence, Gandhi pursued and won independence for his country. The fact that he acquired this mantra from his nurse rather than from an esteemed teacher illustrates an important point: Ultimately, the power of any mantra derives from the sincerity and devotion of those who practice it.

Gandhi chanted this mantra daily for his entire life. At the moment of his death, he could be heard muttering "Hey Ram." In India, it is a traditional aspiration to remember one's chosen spiritual ideal at the end of life. In Vedic writings, this is called the Law of the Last Thought, and it is said to have great importance in determining the next incarnation. As he died, Gandhi was concentrating on his spiritual truth. Perhaps rebirth was not required in his case.

10

Mantras for Abundance and Prosperity

In chapter 9 we touched on the idea that abundance is in the mind of the beholder. Our unique needs, values, hopes, and fears define what abundance means to each of us. And these individual traits, in turn, are defined by the culture in which we live.

The use of healing mantras originated in agrarian societies, where abundance sometimes meant simply having something to eat. While most of us live in relative comfort on the material level, we do have spiritual needs that must be fulfilled. For a child growing up in a home ridden with conflict and abuse, peace and harmony represent genuine abundance. An elderly person, isolated in a rapidly changing world, finds abundance in the companionship of someone who shares the same memories. For the physically disabled, friendship based upon who you are rather than what you can do constitutes yet another form of abundance.

Intention and Procedure

Because the definition of abundance is such an individual matter, your intentions in using mantras for abundance are extremely important. Mantra will always cause the chakras to become energized, but how the energy manifests in your mind and body is determined by the powerful directives you form as conscious and subconscious intentions. The authors of the ancient texts understood this very well, and they instruct us to identify our desires clearly in order to achieve the desired result.

I often suggest that my students write the result they desire on a piece of paper, fold it carefully, and place it in the location where they will most often say the mantra. You can still say the mantra elsewhere: while driving to work, for example, or doing household chores. But I recommend at least one meditation each day in your chosen spot. During this time, focus your thoughts on your individual definition of abundance before you begin. Gradually your particular aspiration will kick in automatically whenever you say the mantra—but it will only do so if you've created this relationship between stimulus and response. So it's extremely important to establish exactly what abundance means to you from the very beginning of the mantra discipline.

Mantras in certain categories, such as health and healing, seem surprisingly general in translation. This is also true of mantras for abundance, such as those below. Once again, if you're able, it's best to use these in a discipline of concentrated meditation for ten to twenty minutes each day over a period of forty days.

The Foundation Abundance Mantra

Because the Vedic and other Eastern traditions routinely describe power in feminine terms, it's not surprising that the foundation mantra for abundance enlists feminine energy.

Om Shrim Maha Lakshmiyei Swaha

(OM SHREEM MAH-HA LAHKSH-MEE-YEI SWAH-HA)

Om, you may remember, is the seed sound for the sixth chakra, where masculine and feminine energies meet at the center of the brow. Because *Om* represents a conjunction of will and sound, it is commonly used as a prefix to mantras of all kinds. Of the millions of mantras that have originated in the Far East over the past five thousand years, more than 95 percent begin with *Om*.

Shrim is the seed sound for the principle of abundance, which is personified by the goddess Lakshmi in the Hindu pantheon. She is often depicted sitting or standing on a lotus flower, beautiful beyond measure, with a stream of coins flowing from her hand. Behind the goddess, elephants are playing, with their trunks upraised. Elephants are a traditional symbol of good fortune, and the raised trunks indicate a propensity to retain the good fortune, rather than spilling it onto the ground.

Maha means "great." In this context it denotes both quantity and quality. When we speak of the quality of abundance here, we are referring to its harmony with dharma or divine law. Abundance of any other kind is more of a burden than a blessing. Imagine, for example, that someone presents you with a large amount of money. Now you have abundant financial resources—but if the money has been stolen you could be implicated in the crime. The prefix *Maha* is intended to prevent this kind of difficulty.

Lakshmi, again, is the principle of abundance. This goddess is such a powerful feminine force that continued use of her Sanskrit name generates great creative energy. But in the simplest terms, she is the personification of wealth. She holds aloft the torch of prosperity in all its forms and for all beings.

Swaha, in this context, means "I salute." It is also related to the manifestation of energy at the solar plexus chakra. Mantras exist in masculine, feminine, and neutral forms. Here, *Swaha* provides a feminine ending.

This mantra can be used to attain abundance in almost any form. If you're able, commit yourself to a forty-day program. It's best to set aside thirty minutes or so each day to chant quietly by yourself. At other times, say the mantra as often as possible.

When you face a problem related to abundance, remember that the general nature of the mantra will immediately help the chakras to begin processing new levels of energy. The kundalini will start to send out energy related to the principle you are invoking with your mantra.

You will be drawing in energy from your spiritual surroundings, but you must also focus your mental efforts to have a clear understanding of that which is desired. As the saying goes, "Be careful what you ask for, you just might get it."

A Personal Example

After twenty-five years of working with mantra almost exclusively for spiritual ends, I had not used mantra specifically to gain prosperity. Even though mantra had once helped me find a job, believe it or not, it just never occurred to me to use mantra for material gain . . . until one day when things began to get tight financially. Then I decided that I had better practice what I'd been teaching about achieving prosperity.

I used the foundation mantra given above. I also kept a daily diary of how many repetitions I completed each day. I decided to perform the classical forty-day discipline. I used a small notebook for both my statement of need and a record of my work with mantra.

I work with mantra for hours at a time. It has become such a well-integrated part of my life that I can center myself in a mantra and go about my daily activities in quite a normal way. Part of me, however, is constantly at work with some mantra. For this prosperity discipline, the mantra was the *Maha Lakshmiyei.*

After I'd been working with the mantra for a week, some friends called and said that they had a booth at the Whole Life Expo in San Francisco and they would be happy to share it with me if I wanted to sell my books and tapes. Margalo and I packed our bags and boxes of books and headed off to the Expo. Over the next three days I sold many books and tapes. I continued to do my mantra. Upon my return, I found that sales from my Web site had picked up dramatically. I had to do new print runs of all my materials to keep up with the demand. At the conclusion of the forty-day discipline I had chanted the mantra many, many times, and I felt that the results would continue, as they often do when you have completed the mantra discipline in a very focused way.

Within a short time after the completion of the discipline, a client for whom I was doing consulting work wanted me to come in much more frequently. After several months of increased activity, he asked me to come on retainer for an amount that would well serve my needs. Also around that time, I found a new literary agent who liked my books, and I sold the very book you are now reading. So, for me, the mantra discipline worked extremely powerfully. It can work powerfully for you as well.

Please remember that Lakshmi includes spiritual abundance as well as physical plane abundance. Compassion, sympathy, empathy, maternal love, the fire of maternal protection, and a constant and effortless flow of spiritual wisdom backed by divine authority are all included within the Lakshmi principle.

A Mantra for Children

Om Namo Bhagavate Vasudevaya

(OM NAH-MO BHAH-GAH-VAH-TEH VAH-SOO-DAY-VAH-YAH)

This is the great twelve-syllable mantra that is widely practiced by many diverse Hindu sects in India. It is known as a Mukti, or liberation, mantra. Although their philosophic approach to truth or realization may be widely divergent, all those who use the mantra recognize the potency of this spiritual formula.

Consistent use of this mantra will eventually free us from the cycle of rebirth. Repeated trips to this planet for the purpose of paying off karma will become unnecessary. Each of us crosses the ocean of this samsara, the ceaselessly tossing ocean of innumerable causes and effects of the inhabitants of this universe. These, collectively, create the totality of karma in the realms of existence we experience before, during, and after birth in a particular body. The meaning of liberation from rebirth is real freedom of choice. But this mantra can be applied in another context, which is related to its meaning. Paradoxically, while this mantra can free your own spirit from repeated negative patterns of rebirth or behavior in this life, it can also help you prepare the way for the life of another soul, a child's.

Vasudeva is the individual Indweller aspect of God. The word invokes the connection of the soul, the Indweller, with the omnipresence of three qualities of existence: Sat (truth or existence), Chit (spiritual mind stuff), and Ananda (bliss), as they exist throughout creation. This connection brings the sublime qualities of consciousness into a specific form: a specific body, a specific person.

Om is the prefix. It is a seed sound for the sixth, or brow, chakra, where the feminine and masculine currents meet. *Om* is the name of the state of existence in which the individual Indweller (jiva, atman, or soul) has united with the all-pervading divine substance, the spirit of God.

Namo, here, means "name," or more specifically, "name of."

Bhagavate is a specific individual who is now in the process of becoming divine. It can be either a person now born or an already spiritually developed soul. One offers to bring such a soul into physical-place embodiment.

Vasudevaya is "the Indweller." The divine substance, giver of all, knower of all, apart but not separate from the divine substance everywhere.

This is a somewhat complicated but fairly complete meaning for the energy of the mantra. Sanskrit is primarily an energy-based language rather than a meaning-based one. A much more universally acknowledged surface meaning for the mantra is, "Om and salutations to the Indwelling One, substance of the Divine."

As you can see, the "Indwelling One" can also refer to a baby. In the spiritual stories surrounding Krishna, Vasudeva was his father, which provides another hidden pointer to using this mantra for bringing a spiritual person into a physical body as your child. So if you desire a child, and especially if you want a child for spiritual reasons such as helping to make a conscious contribution to this world, perform a classical forty-day spiritual discipline with this mantra and focus on the spiritual intentions you have for your baby. In so doing, you will help us all.

It's a Boy

About twenty years ago some friends of mine wanted to have a spiritually inclined baby. The sex of the child did not matter. To achieve this end they were given a mantra by an Indian teacher we all knew at the time. The mantra was *Om Namo Bhagavate Vasudevaya.*

The couple meditated together and completed a forty-day discipline of the mantra. Soon, Barbara conceived and the couple was of course very happy. At the third month, there was an incident where she thought she'd had a spontaneous abortion. All of their friends and family were disappointed and everyone consoled the couple.

Yet after another six weeks, Barbara began to feel that she was pregnant. She went to the doctor and found she was in her fourth month. She had not lost the baby at all. She went on to have a healthy and happy boy named William.

An Experiment

One aspect of the doctrine of reincarnation teaches that children, and particularly babies, are more in touch with their divine nature than adults. As we become acculturated, we forget our previous lives.

I decided to use my friendship with William's parents, with whom I lived at the Center, to conduct my own experiment that would test whether or not William could make contact with a past life. I waited for the right moment, which came when he was no more than eight months old. I decided that the best way to test William would be to present him with certain classical spiritual stimuli and see if I got any reaction at all. My experiment was to "recognize" the divinity in William by giving him a common Far Eastern spiritual salute.

One day when I entered the house, William's parents were in the kitchen preparing food. William himself was in a baby carrier on one of the kitchen counters. He was facing the back door, where I entered. As I came in, I placed my palms together in front of my heart in the *namaste* spiritual greeting and bowed my head ever so slightly toward him. The baby immediately gurgled happily, stretched forth his tiny hand, and formed an ancient mudra, or divine gesture. This was the *jnana* mudra, or gesture of wisdom. The *jnana* mudra is made by joining the thumb and first finger on the right hand, with the thumb slightly extended beyond the tip of the first finger, and the other three fingers joined together. It looks a little like the "OK" sign we give to one another. However, in the *jnana* mudra, the arm is extended and the hand raised at the wrist, with the palm pointing toward the person to whom the mudra is aimed. William performed this ancient mudra perfectly. The hair on my head stood on end and goose pimples rose on my arms in waves. I looked at the baby, momentarily stunned. The baby looked back at me with complete conscious awareness, recognition, and intelligence. It was not the look of an infant.

Suddenly one of the parents turned around with a bottle. The moment was over. William was given the bottle and began to suck vigorously. I came over and looked at the baby closely. I got his attention and looked into his eyes. There was only an infant glancing fleetingly and vacantly at me. William's attention was utterly absorbed in the bottle. I tried to tell the parents about the moment. They were pleased that I said special things about their baby, but they, too, were distracted and really had no interest in "the moment." I realized that this experiment was strictly for me, but it was enough.

A Mantra for Gaining Friends and Companions

There is an old saying that the best way to get love is by giving love to others. Similarly, if we want friends and companions, being a good friend to others is a good way to begin. There is a mantra for producing the quality of friendship in oneself. The mantra is one of the "twelve great qualities of the sun."

Om Hraum Mitraya Namaha

(OM HROUWM MEE-TRAH-YAH NAHM-AH-HA)

The intention of this mantra is the creation of friendship in a very special sense: when you become a friend to everyone, everyone will view you as a friend.

Removing Obstacles to Prosperity

There are times when efforts, even those from powerful mantras, seem not to be working as we wanted or as we think they should. It is as if some obstacle or barrier is in the way.

Ganesha's mantra, discussed in chapter 5, is the quintessential obstacle remover.

Om Gum Ganapatayei Namaha

(OM GUM GUH-NUH-PUH-TUH-YEI NAHM-AH-HA)

*"Om and salutations to the remover of
obstacles for which Gum is the seed."*

11

===

Mantras for Self-empowerment

High school geometry courses teach that, from even a small segment of a circle, you can infer the circumference, diameter, area, and all other vital information pertaining to the figure. Just a few centimeters of perfectly curved line provides all the information necessary to accurately arrive at characteristics of the circle it indicates. Since 1973, I have experimented with mantras for a variety of conditions and circumstances. The experience gained over those years represents a few centimeters of perfectly curved line: I know that mantras work, and work powerfully.

This chapter provides mantras you can use to gain power for the pursuit of your spiritual, creative, educational, and professional goals.

Mantra for Confidence and Inner Strength

From time to time I am approached by people, particularly women, who profess a lack of self-confidence. In such cases, I always recommend the following mantra. In fact, I wish I could give this mantra to every woman who has doubts about her own abilities or her own power. Associated with the feminine principle, this mantra produces an extremely powerful effect, giving a sense of one's power and the wisdom to use that power wisely.

Om Eim Hrim Klim Chamundayei
Vichei Namaha

(OM I'M HREEM KLEEM CHAH-MOON-DAH-YEI
VEE-CHEH NAHM-AH-HA)

*"Om and salutations to she who is radiant
with power and wisdom."*

Om is the seed of unity of feminine and masculine energies at the
brow center. *Eim* is the seed sound for Saraswati, who presides over
sound, the arts, and science both spiritual and material. This energy is
also associated with dispelling certain types of negative energy. *Hrim*
(as before) is a seed sound for dissolving the appearance of reality.
Klim (as before) is a seed sound for attraction. *Chamunda[i]* is a beautiful aspect of the feminine which, nonetheless, can be utterly destructive to a wide variety of negative forces and influences. *Yei* is
a Shakti-activating sound. *Namaha* has previously been discussed in
detail.

As with many mantras, the effects produced by saying this one
vary according to the user. One woman reported that this mantra produced a feeling of joy so intense that she did not want to stop reciting
it. Another person told me that it filled him with a sense of power.
Please remember, if you recite the mantra for a long period of time
during a single day or for many days and begin to feel any discomfort,
stop your practice for a few hours or days and let your prana readjust to
the new vibration level you are creating.

Good-Luck Mantra

Like Ganesha, the god invoked in this mantra is a son of Shiva and Parvati. Whereas Ganesha is very close to his mother, and thus associated with an almost primal power, Skanda (or Kartikeya—he goes by several names) is more associated with Shiva and consciousness, which may also act as a directed force. Here, the individual consciousness is imbued with strength, optimism, and auspiciousness. These conditions seem to produce "good luck" or a general good outcome from a variety of circumstances.

Om Sharavana Bhavaya Namaha

(OM SHAH-RAH-VAH-NAH BHAH-VAH-YAH NAHM-AH-HA)

"Om and salutations to the son of Shiva, who brings auspiciousness and who is chief of the celestial army."

Spiritual Growth

There are many mantras that can help your spiritual growth and insight. One is:

Om Nama Shivaya

(OM NAH-MAH SHEE-VAH-YAH)

This Siddha mantra uses the universal elements that govern each chakra: earth, water, fire, air, and ether. The syllables *Na, Ma, Shi, Va,* and *Ya* help the chakras to better utilize the fundamental elements that predominate in the chakra. One who is a siddha is a perfected being. This mantra leads you powerfully toward spiritual maturity. Thus, this mantra is from the tradition of the path of Perfection of the Divine Vehicle, which refers to the human body in all of its gross and subtle parts.

Mantra for Destruction of Negative Forces and for Protection

This is a mantra for the avatar of Vishnu known as Narasimha. A composite spiritual being with aspects of humanity, divinity, and animal nature all mixed together, this avatar defeated a supposedly unconquerable one of great evil. While the mantra invokes powerful energy, one's righteous internal attitude provides a buffer against misusing it. This mantra can backfire if used in a hateful way, because hate is contrary to the nature of all Vishnu mantras.

Narasimha Ta Va Da So Hum

(NAH-RAH-SEEM-HA TAH VAH DAH SOH HUHM)

Narasimha is the principle for destroying the seemingly indestructible. *Ta* is the seed sound (without "m") of the lower leg from the knee to the ankle. *Va* is the seed (without "m" of the second chakra) for the genital center. *Da* is a sound for directing the energy for the highest good. *So Hum* brings the mind in tune with the divine self within.

According to Vedic lore, whenever evil influences rule the earth an incarnation of the Divine will arrive to save humanity. Narasimha was one such incarnation. It seems there was an evil ruler who was so powerful that he could not possibly be defeated in battle. It was said that "He could not be defeated during the day or the night. Nor by man nor beast. Nor could he be defeated either indoors or outdoors."

Vishnu, in mercy and compassion, came to earth as Narasimha, a man-lion being. Narasimha sought out the evil tyrant's dwelling place and waited. At twilight, he entered, found the tyrant, and dragged him to the threshold. Holding him firmly, Narasimha began to speak: "It is twilight, neither day nor night. It is on the threshold of your dwelling, neither inside nor outdoors. I am neither man nor beast, but a combination of both. Therefore, I now destroy you." And he ripped the evil tyrant into pieces.

From that time to this, Narasimha has been invoked to gain freedom from evil situations.

A friend of mine named Frank came to me concerned that a relative was attempting to gain undue influence over his father, who was dying. The relative seemed bent on gaining as much of the sizable inheritance as possible. After meditating upon the problem for a few moments, I recommended saying the Narasimha mantra below, at the rate of a minimum of five hundred repetitions per day. I told him a thousand repetitions per day would be better, if he could manage it. The discipline was undertaken every day, with five hundred repetitions completed some days and a thousand repetitions chanted on other days. The inheritance issue was equitably settled for all family members when Frank's father passed away several months later.

Sikh Mantra for Spiritual Advancement

Sikhism is a union of principles from Hinduism and Islam. Followers of this religion are welcome in almost any culture because of their dedication to hard work and the improvement of the community in which they reside. This includes Islamic countries where very few outside religions are tolerated. Sikhism is, therefore, unique in its universal

acceptance among various cultures and countries. This mantra invokes
the energy of the Inner Teacher and contact with the Great Ones of
their religion who have come before.

Ek Ong Kar Sat Nam Siri Wahe Guru

(EK ONG KAR SAHT NAHM SEE-REE WHA-HEI GOO-ROO)

*"There is One Creator who has created this creation. Truth is His
name. He is so great we cannot describe His infinite wisdom."*

Spiritual Advancement Using Masculine and Feminine Energy

The following mantra is closely associated with the breath. It is written
in some of the ancient texts that *So Hum* is the subtle sound of the
breath itself.

So Hum

(SOH-HUHM)

When the autonomic nervous system becomes conscious instead
of operating unconsciously, the mantra changes to *Hum So*.

Om Hum So Hum

(OM HUHM SOH HUHM)

There is no real translation for this mantra. It is concerned with energy, breath, and the placement of consciousness. It is one of the simplest and yet most powerful mantras for permanently altering your state of consciousness. It balances the masculine and feminine energies and focuses their combined force.

Mantra for Compassion

This mantra invokes Shiva in a compassionate feminine form, closely related to Durga.

Sarva Mangala Mangalyei
Shive Sarvartha Sadikei
Sharanyei Tryambakei Gauri
Narayani Namostute

(SAHR-VAH MAHN-GAH-LAH MAHN-GAHL-YEI

SHEE-VEI SAHR-VARH-TAH SAH-DEE-KEI

SHAH-RAHN-YEI TRAH-YAHM-BAH-KEH GOW-REE

NAH-RAH-YAN-NEE NAH-MOH-STOO-TEH)

"Oh Great Feminine power which is the driving energy of Shiva, Narayana, whose very touch brings ecstasy, one who opens the eye of wisdom, bestow upon us the highest blessings."

Mangala means "one whose touch brings ecstasy." *Shive, Tryambake,* and *Gauri* are all feminine forms of beings that are usually shown in masculine representation. *Narayani* is a feminine representation (in this case, sister) of Narayana, lord of the threefold flame that can manifest anything at will, including entire universes.

Mantra for Spiritual Insight

Chant this mantra, for Brahma the Creator to achieve understanding of the mysteries of the form of creation. Through the chanting of this mantra, the secrets of the Universe become accessible to you.

Sat Chid Ekam Brahma

(SAHT CHEED EH-KAHM BRAH-MAH)

Here is what the various words mean in their energy context: *Sat:* Truth; *Chid:* Spiritual mind-stuff; *Ekam:* One, without a second; *Brahma:* This entire cosmos, with all of its contents.

This is also a longer version of the *Sat Chid Ekam Brahma* mantra:

Om Eim Hrim Shrim Klim Sauh Sat Chid Ekam Brahma

(OM I'M HREEM SHREEM KLEEM SAW

SAHT CHEED EH-KAM BRAH-MAH)

Om is a prefix to many mantras. It represents the energy at the Ajna chakra at the brow center, where the feminine and masculine currents become joined and consciousness becomes unitary and holistic.

Eim is a seed sound for the feminine principle known as Saraswati. This principle governs spiritual knowledge as well as the material pursuits of education, science, art, music, and spiritual discipline.

Hrim is a seed sound for Mahamaya, or the veil of creation. It is said that meditation on this seed sound will result in the meditator ultimately being shown the universe "as it is" and not as we see it currently. That is because reality as we see it is really an "agreement" among all of us that is passed on from generation to generation. Babies, if they could talk, would speak of the universe in quite a different way. They ultimately learn what humanity's "agreement" is and start to function in the world.

Shrim is the seed sound for the principle of abundance. This covers the abundance of food, friends, family, health, and myriad other things. Prosperity is, of course, included.

Klim is a seed with several meanings. In the present context, it is the principle of attraction. In this mantra, it is attracting the fruit of the other principles to speed the process of mantra meditation.

Sauh is a spiritual principle that operates through one of the petals in the Ajna chakra. It is also a Shakti-activating sound.

Hanuman Mantras for Healing Energy (Prana) and Athletic Strength

In stories about the avatar Rama, Hanuman is depicted as the perfect servant. The life of Rama recorded in the *Ramayana*, with versions by poets Valmiki and Tulasidas, provides an allegory for the spiritual development of humankind that is eloquent and poetic. Here, in brief, is what happened to Rama and the esoteric significance of those events.

Rama is the Divine Self. Sita is the perfect and pure kundalini

shakti. As eldest son, Rama is destined to rule the kingdom when King
Dasaratha dies, but through court intrigue the king is forced to appoint
Rama's brother Bharata (the mind) to the throne. Rama is to be banished to the forest for twelve years. Bharata knows that false deeds had
led to Rama's banishment and has placed Rama's sandals (the power of
the Self manifesting through kundalini) on the throne and declared
him to be the true king, in exile or not. Bharata then declares that he
will act as Rama's steward until his return, and that Rama's sandals
upon the throne will demonstrate to all who the true ruler is.

The mind must always act as a steward for the Divine. For the divinity within is the Self, located at the heart center, and not the mind,
which has no light of its own.

Sita is subsequently abducted by Ravana, the last of the evil kings,
and taken a great distance away. Ravana wants Sita to become his consort. He is driven by lustful desires devoid of any love or true feeling
whatever.

Meanwhile Rama is traveling in the forest, where he happens
upon Hanuman (the prana), a chief of one of the monkey tribes. Hanuman pledges his allegiance to Rama and becomes his foremost servant. Rama sends Hanuman in search of Sita.

Selfish and egotistical desires have appropriated the divine energy
within. The kundalini shakti is prevented from joining the Divine Self
located at the heart center, and is detained at the second chakra (lust
and magical powers) and the third chakra (dominion over the elements
of earth, water, and fire, as well as temporal desires of all kinds). But
Hanuman, representing the prana, is sent to find Sita. This is the
practice of the rhythmic breathing the yogi employs to purify the
body and chakras, and bring the kundalini up to the heart center and
beyond.

Hanuman finds Ravana and his brother Kumbarnaka and a huge
battle ensues. Since Hanuman is not powerful enough to defeat Ravana, he cannot liberate Sita. But neither can Hanuman be defeated.
He returns to Rama and tells him where Sita is detained.

The pranic breathing will always disclose the location of the kundalini and where its energy may be held captive.

Rama and Lakshmana go to the realm of Ravana and Kumbarnaka and do battle with them. When they finally confront one another, Rama reveals his divine nature, and Ravana melts into praise and becomes a devotee, with tears of devotion streaming from his eyes.

The Divine can change even the vilest of us into a repository of divine virtues in an instant of blessing. Individually, even in parts of us where the most disgusting or egocentric karma may be stored, the stainless nature of the Divine Self can melt that karma away in an instant.

Rama and Sita return from the forest and their coronation takes place on a grand scale.

The spirit and the soul, when finally united—at first in the heart center and then at the crown chakra—bring us to the apex of the development possible while in human form.

Hanuman mantras work directly with the prana. The more mantra is performed, the more the prana becomes imbued with the consciousness present in the sound and energy of the mantra. This fact alone supports the position of some religious scholars who state that Hanuman is related to the energy of Shiva.

There are two Hanuman mantras that greatly strengthen the prana of any individual or healer who uses them.

Om Hum Hanumate Vijayam

(OM HOOM HAH-NOO-MAH-TEH VEE-JAY-YAHM)

"Victory to the prana in its evolutionary course, as it strengthens the will through the throat center."

For those involved in athletics, this mantra can aid in gaining both strength and agility.

Om Sri Hanumate Namaha

(OM SHREE HAH-NOO-MAH-TEH NAHM-AH-HA)

"Salutations to the conscious prana."

With this mantra, healers strengthen their ability to transfer healing prana to their patients.

Saraswati Mantras for Knowledge and Creative Achievement

Shown holding a stringed instrument in one hand and a mala in the other, with a book at her feet, Saraswati is a feminine power that activates and sustains artistic, academic, and spiritual endeavors. Eastern artists and musicians practice Saraswati japa (recitation of mantra). Mothers chant Saraswati japa on behalf of their children to help them do well in school. Spiritual teachers chant Saraswati japa to obtain the capacity to hold the highest wisdom. Teachers, secular and spiritual, chant Saraswati japa to ensure that the words coming out of their mouths contain the truth and the correct principles desired. They want to be persuasive to their hearers. All this is the province of Saraswati.

Saraswati is one of the Hindu feminine trinity of Lakshmi, Durga, and Saraswati. But her power is least talked about in the West. We hear much about Lakshmi's gifts of abundance and Durga's provisions of protection, but much less about Saraswati. Why should this be? It may be that most knowledgeable spiritual teachers from the Far East want to keep "true spiritual knowledge" secret, and Saraswati is the path to that knowledge.

In the earliest Vedic writings, Saraswati is referred to as Vach, the goddess of speech in the primordial sense—that is, the source of all speech, both divine and mundane. She represents:

- The sacrificial word, the primal cause, and the mystical "name" referred to by the Kabbalists;
- The power, mistress, and constructor of mantra;
- The goddess of hidden wisdom.

There is an old and ongoing "divine disputation" to determine which is superior, mind or speech. The final answer in this discussion is that ultimately mind is superior, but only after the realm of creation has been left behind. The "catch" is that the realm of creation includes all of the subtle realms wherein masters and all the celestials in all the spheres may dwell. Mind assumes preeminence only when we withdraw our consciousness from the akashic realm accessible through the Vishuddha Chakra at the throat center and travel to the place where duality ends.

The significance of Saraswati for today's practitioner of mantra can be summed up in a few points. The Saraswati energy, according to the ancient scriptures:

- Governs all spiritual pursuits;
- Gives mantras their power—spiritual teachers and gurus transmit the power of mantra through the Saraswati energy;
- Rules followers of the path of intellectual understanding and mind;
- Governs the transmission of a powerful shakti, or energy of transformation, as recorded by many famous teachers such as Yogananda and Ramakrishna;
- Is adopted by many Himalayan adepts and swamis as part of their spiritual name.

Mantra for Success in Education, Music, and Artistic Endeavors.

Om Eim Saraswatiyei Swaha

(OM I'M SAH-RAH-SWAH-TEE-YEI SWAH-HA)

"Om and salutations to the feminine Saraswati principle."

In any creative endeavor, this mantra invokes energy for making the project fruitful and successful.

Maha Vidya: Queen of Knowledge Mantra.

Eim Hrim Srim Klim Sauh Klim Hrim Eim Blum Strim Nilatari Saraswati Dram Drim Klim Blum Sah Eim Hrim Srim Klim Sauh Sauh Hrim Swaha

(I'M HREEM SHREEM KLEEM SAW KLEEM HREEM I'M
BLOOM STREEM NEE-LAH-TAH-REE SAH-RAH-SWAH-TEE
DRAHM DREEM KLEEM BLOOM SAW I'M HREEM SHREEM
KLEEM SAW SAW HREEM SWAH-HA)

This Saraswati "freight train" mantra is a succession of seed mantras and is therefore essentially untranslatable. Faithful repetition of this mantra will, over time, transform the sayer into a person of great spiritual knowledge.

Mantra for Seeing the Self Within and the Universe as One

Narayana is the inner eternal flame located in the Hrit Padma, or "sacred heart," an eight-petaled secret chakra two finger-widths below the heart center. It manifests according to one's devotion. This single attribute accounts for wonderful and fulfilling experiences for genuine seekers on the one hand, and for tremendous confusion on the other.

In the Narayanaya Suktam it is said that Narayana is Brahma, Vishnu, and Siva. It is the light dwelling in the sacred heart that conforms to the devotion of each person. Thus, when Narayana manifests, it is as the person's chosen ideal. This causes confusion, because different people have different chosen ideals. The experience of a divine vision of the Beloved is so powerful that the experiencer believes the experience is absolute instead of relative. One person may see Krishna and another, Jesus. The confusion arises because not *every* divine experience of these beings is authentic in the sense of a real visitation. Sometimes it is the sacred heart manifesting due to the intense devotion of the person.

Om Namo Narayanaya takes the sayer to sublime spiritual realms where spiritual questions are answered and great truths are revealed. Spiritual encounters with the Divine Beloved can be positively life-transforming. Actual sages from antiquity who are dwelling in the subtle realms may appear and instruct. Desires may suddenly be fulfilled. This mantra is both wonderful and mysterious.

In India there is a universal truth ceremony called Satya Narayana Puja. People from many castes and creeds practice this ceremony. It cuts across and through sectarian differences and preferences. Hence it is regarded as universal.

Om Namo Narayanaya

(OM NAH-MOH NAH-RAH-YAH-NAY-YAH)

"Om is the Name of Narayana, the flame of truth."

Mantra for Divine Guidance on the Spiritual Path

This last mantra is sung at the conclusion of various kinds of religious ceremonies derived from the Vedic tradition. One can hear it exactly the same way in India, Trinidad, or the Philippines. It is my prayer for us all as well.

Om Asatoma Sad Gamaya
Tamasoma Jyothir Gamaya
Mrityorma Umritam Gamaya
Om Shanti, Shanti, Shantihi

(OM AH-SAH-TOH-MAH SAHD GAH-MAH-YAH

TAH-MAH-SOH-MAH JYOH-TEER GAH-MAH-YAH

MRIT-YOHR-MAH AHM-REE-TAHM GAH-MAH-YAH

OM SHAHN-TEE SHAHN-TEE SHAHN-TEE-HEE)

"Lead us from unreality to reality
From darkness to light
From death to immortality
Om peace, peace, peace."

12

Chanting for the Planet

All of us are aware that the world has problems. Most of us have thought, "I wish I could do something to help humanity come to its senses." Many of us pray daily, and that has helped us all, I am sure. Even so, more can always be done. For those who want to do something different from prayer and in addition to community service, this chapter will provide a path for helping the planet through mantra. The idea of chanting for the planet came to me through an extraordinary event in my life.

Throwing His Voice

Whenever my friend Dr. Charles Wesley called me, I paid attention. Charles had been on the spiritual path for all of his adult life, practicing meditations learned from various teachers and adapted for his own uses for nearly forty years. At the time of this story, I, on the other hand, was a relative newcomer with only five years of meditation background. So, when Charles recommended that I go to the Tibetan Black Hat ceremony at Georgetown University that evening, I determined that I would go. This special ceremony is performed only by the Karma-pa who is the head of the Karma Kagyu branch of Tibetan Buddhism.

The large hall on the main campus of Georgetown University

holds around three thousand people. A narrow balcony circles the auditorium, which has a stage at the front.

The huge, deep burgundy drape hanging fifty feet down near the front of the stage blended perfectly with the Tibetan motif of the monks and their paraphernalia. I had never seen anything like the long, curved musical horns behind which the monks stood, or the seat for the Sixteenth Gyalwa Karma-pa that was elevated four and a half feet. The elevated seat would give the Tibetan spiritual leader a place to work during the evening ceremony, which was just a few minutes off.

I was seated in row seven in front. This was very good luck, to my way of thinking. I had a really good view of what was going on. Pulling out the program that had been pressed into my hand, I began to read about the Black Hat ceremony.

Several hundred years ago, a local Tibetan monarch had a vivid dream in which he saw the presiding Karma-pa of that time holding a jewel-encrusted black hat. It looked something like a small elevated tent but had rigid curved surfaces instead of windblown fabric. In the dream, the Karma-pa placed the hat on his head and went into an altered state of consciousness, blessing everyone who witnessed it. When the monarch awakened, he called his craftsmen together, made a sketch of what he had seen, and commissioned the creation of the hat seen in his dream. Several attempts later, they finally had it right. The monarch journeyed several days to the monastery of the spiritual leader. The Karma-pa nodded, pulled out a crystal rosary, and placed the hat upon his head. He was immediately transformed by a dazzling light that surrounded him completely. He began to chant the well-known mantra *Om Mani Padme Hum*, which, roughly translated, means "The jewel of consciousness is in the heart's lotus." Everyone who was present went into an exalted state. At that moment, the Black Hat ceremony was born.

Thereafter, all of the succeeding Karma-pas inherited the black hat. At times of their choosing during their lifetime, they would perform the ceremony. They would place the black hat on their head, take a clear crystal rosary, and chant the *"Mani"* 108 times.

When I read that the ceremony involved mantra, I realized why Charles had called me. He knew my spiritual habits well. He had also suggested that we meet after the ceremony. Since he was probably somewhere in the hall, I was vaguely wondering if I could get a ride home from him and avoid a long bus ride.

All of a sudden there was a blare of unimaginable loudness. I looked up and saw that three monks in burgundy and gold robes were blowing into those long horns, which produced a unique racket in prolonged bursts. The more I listened, the less the sound disconcerted me. It seemed almost musical. But my frame of reference for "music" was changing by the second.

Just as I was integrating the sound of the horns into my experience, a slightly potbellied Tibetan man strode purposefully out onto the stage and looked around. The audience applauded. He smiled and, elevating his glance ever so slightly, took a deep diaphragmatic breath. I was seized by the thought that he had just "breathed in" the entire population of the hall in some profound way.

The man climbed three hidden steps to the elevated seat and arranged himself. This took only a few seconds, but I watched his every move to catch each detail. I felt that if I watched him in the right way, I would learn something of great value.

Once seated, he picked up various implements of ceremonial worship and inspected them. Then about twenty other monks joined him onstage. They sat on the floor. Loud sonorous chanting filled the hall with the tones and resonances uniquely characteristic of Tibetan chanting. I began to feel myself relaxing in some deep way. At the same time, my awareness became heightened. I observed carefully as various items were used in a ceremony that unfolded over a period of thirty minutes. Then a large, ornate hat box was pulled out from somewhere and opened. A black hat studded with what looked like diamonds emerged from the interior, and the Karma-pa placed it on his head and pulled out a clear crystal rosary. The whole group began to chant *Om Mani Padme Hum*, and the chanting went on for a few minutes.

I noticed that the minute the Karma-pa placed the hat upon his head, his face changed. He looked twenty years younger and his countenance seemed to glow.

Unexpectedly, the ceremony ended and a line formed at the left side of the stage steps. Since my row was up front, we were ushered to the front of the line. Each person passed by the elevated chair of the Karma-pa. He spent a moment with each one.

Within a few minutes, it was my turn. I stood there not knowing what to do. He calmly reached down and pulled my head forward until it was bent over in front of him. He placed a warm metal object on the nape of my neck and chanted. Then I looked up, dazed, and he smiled very, very sweetly and showed me a picture the size of a playing card. I hadn't the faintest idea who the monk in the picture was. Still don't. Then the moment was over and I was receiving a piece of red thread and a handful of multicolored rice, and I was out of the line and back on the floor of the hall. I had no idea what any of it was about.

I decided to look for Charles from the balcony. I began the tedious task of weaving my way through the crowd to the stairs leading up, taking about ten agonizing minutes to get there. Once I reached the stairs, I quickly got to the top, and among a handful of people, there was Charles. I waved but he didn't see me. I walked over to where he was standing, seemingly lost in thought, and I said, "Hi, Charles. How lucky to find you in this crowd." He said not a word. Instead, he looked vacantly past me and over toward the stairs. I again said, "Charles!" No response at all. I immediately felt very strange, and a few people started looking at me appraisingly. I took a few steps backward and stood watching Charles. He remained in his place for a full two minutes; then he whirled around and headed for the stairs. I felt I was in a twilight zone.

As I stood there wondering what to do next, all of a sudden there was a clear, booming voice in my chest chanting *Om Mani Padme Hum* over and over again. The voice was audible only to me, and it was, internally, VERY LOUD. It was the loudest thing I have ever heard that did not make a sound.

I think my mouth dropped open. I just stood still and experienced it. Then I was seized by an inspiration.

I strode over to the railing at the front of the balcony and looked straight at the Karma-pa some sixty yards away. He was still seeing individuals in the line that snaked around the hall for hundreds of yards. I looked at him, and I mentally shouted at him, "Is this you?" He immediately jerked his head up and looked directly at me. He beamed an absolutely infectious grin at me and then bent down, continuing his work. I was flabbergasted. And filled with joy.

I stood there, trying not to attract attention to myself. I was afraid someone would come up to me and say that I had to "come with them" or that one of the monks would confront me with interrupting the Karma-pa at work, or something. But I felt absolutely terrific. I was radiating. The chanting in my chest continued for maybe another five minutes ... which is a long, long time ... and then it abruptly stopped. I hurried to catch the next bus home.

Later I confronted Charles with my story and asked him what his experience was. He looked at me quizzically and said, "What experience?" I told him about how he had not seen me in the balcony and how I had been unable to get his attention. He just smiled and shook his head. He hadn't the faintest idea what I was talking about. He'd had a good time, but nothing out of the ordinary had happened. He found my story fascinating but had no memory of seeing me. He believed my experience, but nothing had happened for him except a nice peaceful time. I concluded that the Karma-pa had also put Charles in some strange zone of consciousness where he was mostly oblivious to his surroundings. We joked about that night for years.

Spiritual Initiation

Spiritual initiation may take any number of forms. One of the most classic methods of initiation involves the transmission of a mantra that has been charged with spiritual energy by the initiator. The mantra is then practiced by the newly initiated so that the spiritual charge grows and grows in him or her. I concluded that the Karma-pa had initiated me even though I had never studied with him.

Since mantras can be handed down in this way from one generation to the next, a spiritual lineage is formed. If one asks the right questions, one can trace spiritual lineage back for centuries. All persons in the lineage are connected by a common thread: the mantra.

It is true that mantras will work whether or not one has been initiated because the sounds are directly linked to the activities of the chakras. But it is also true that a mantra charged by a spiritually advanced teacher can significantly cut the time needed for the mantra to have deep-seated spiritual effectiveness.

Ultimately, the mantra transforms the practitioner into a higher state. That state may be dramatically evident or entirely unnoticeable to the people around. Each case is unique. Many great spiritual teachers throughout history have initiated students through mantras.

I saw the Karma-pa a total of three more times: once for the Refuge ceremony, once for the Bodhisattva Vow ceremony, and once more for another Black Hat ceremony three years later. I was on the West Coast two years after that when news of his passing reached me. He may be gone, but the mantra is ever with me.

First Wesak

My experience with the Karma-pa inspired me. Every year, the Birth and Death of the Buddha is celebrated at the full moon when the Sun is in Taurus. This celebration, called the Wesak Festival by Buddhists, usually takes place in May.

I gather with a few friends, and we perform a Wesak ceremony observed by followers of the esoteric Buddhist path, who are more universal in their approach to spirituality. We gather to celebrate the sanctification by the Christ and the Buddha together of all the spiritual work done on the planet Earth during the past year. This includes work performed by all the religious organizations, supplicants, mendicants, seekers, priests, rabbis, monks, masters, mullahs, swamis, students, teachers, disciples, and others working for the redemption of the human soul and the elevation of humanity. We chant mantras from five of the world's great religions. We also chant the *Mani* for from two to twelve hours. We have been doing it since 1975. It has become an annual event to help humanity and the planet through the chanting of mantra.

I organized the first Wesak ceremony at the center in Washington, D.C., in honor of my experience with the Karma-pa. Since then, it has become our tradition to accommodate everyone's different schedule while chanting continuously for several hours. During the period of chanting, people come and go. Some come and chant with us for a few minutes, others for several hours. One year, two women came and chanted for the entire twelve hours we had established for the observance.

During my first Wesak celebration, I had a profound experience. After chanting for about ten hours, I was wiped out. I could not keep awake any longer. But there were still two hours to go in the twelve-hour program, and I wanted to fulfill my self-determined obligation. One of the women who came to the Center frequently could see that I was through. She offered to complete the final two hours and encouraged me to go to bed. I did so with little resistance.

I lay down for a few moments, and suddenly a huge "hole" opened up in my mind's eye. In place of the blackness just before sleep, an opening similar to the iris of a camera appeared and a shaft of light came through it into me. It was unlike any light I have ever seen. It was light of every color: there were greens and oranges, blues and yellows, and other vivid colors. It was dazzling in a sense that is impossible to describe. After a moment of bathing me in light, the iris closed.

I lay there stunned for a moment. Then I remembered the story and the explanation of the Wesak ceremony on the subtle planes.

In a hidden valley, the masters and teachers of the world's great religions gather. At the front of the valley is a large flat rock. On it is a crystal bowl filled with a divine liquid of some sort. As the full moon approaches, the Buddha can be seen descending in a blaze of light. At the exact moment of the full moon, the Christ appears in back of the crystal bowl and intones a mantra known only to him. He touches the bowl and transmits spiritual energy. The mantra is also a signal to the Buddha to release an outpouring of spiritual energy for the planet. That combination of the Buddha and the Christ simultaneously releasing blessings is known as the Great Outpouring.

As I lay there in my bed in the dark, I realized I had received my "piece" of the Great Outpouring. I knew that spiritual people everywhere also get their "piece" of the Outpouring. The experience and the understanding it conveyed were so deeply satisfying that I remind people every year that they should think of it as a part of Easter—a great renewal.

Although I have been a part of many Wesak celebrations since then, nothing compares with the experience of the first one. But it does not matter to me. I have concluded that I was shown something so that I would continue to organize and perform the Wesak celebration. Although I left the Center many years ago, I perform the Wesak every year. Barring the unforeseen, I shall continue to do so as long as I can draw breath.

Traditional and Nontraditional Wesak

Buddhists of all sects all over the world have observed a form of the Wesak ceremony for centuries. On the full moon in May, Buddhist temples receive their congregations, who all celebrate the birth, enlightenment, and death of the Buddha at this time. Sometimes only the monks chant mantras, sometimes everyone present chants, and sometimes there is only meditation. But the object is the same: celebration of the Buddha.

I wanted a Wesak Festival that would honor at least five of the world's religions: Judaism, Christianity, Hinduism, Chinese Buddhism, mainstream Buddhism, and Tibetan Buddhism. I use different branches of Buddhism because that is where the Wesak Festival originated. Selecting a mantra from each tradition, those of us who gather chant each one a minimum of 108 times: one mala, or two rosaries. Most of the mantras are chanted for at least two malas. Then, at the end, the great *Mani* mantra is chanted for at least two hours, sometimes as long as ten hours.

Here are the mantras I have been using for Wesak since 1975:

Hebrew Mantra in Praise of God.

Baruch Atoh Adonai Elohenu Mehloch Aholum

(BAH-ROOK AD-TOH ADD-OH-NEYE EL-OH-HEY-NOO
MAY-LOCK AH-HOH-LUHM)

"Blessed art Thou, O lord our God, King of the universe."

This great Hebrew mantra invokes the almighty lord of the universe. By chanting it for a sustained period of time, one can feel very positive energy accumulating in the solar plexus and the throat chakra. We use this Hebrew chant as the opening invocation for all that follows.

Mantra in Praise of Jesus, Carrying the Authority of the Transcendental Purusha.

Om Jesu Christaya Paramatmane Purusha Avataraya Namaha

(OM YEA-SOO KRIS-TEYE-YAH PAH-RAHM-AHT-MAH-NEH

POO-ROO-SHAH AH-VAH-TAHR-EYE-YAH NAHM-AH-HA)

This mantra states that Jesus is a true world teacher, a presiding soul of all the souls, carrying the authority of the Divine.

Mantra Invoking Vajrapani, the Protector of Dharma and Great Initiator.

Hung Vajra Peh

(HOONG VAHJ-RAH PAY)

Tibetan Buddhism teaches that there is a sphere of consciousness surrounding our planet. Within this sphere are destructive forces that are sometimes called thought-forms. These packages of negative energy created by anger, violence, terrible events (like world wars), and other ignominious aspects of consciousness cause havoc every day. Circulating like blobs of oil within the ocean of consciousness, these bits of gunk need to be neutralized in some way. The Tibetans use the mantra of Vajrapani to disperse these items of consciousness-gunk. In the aspect of protecting the pious and initiating those who qualify, the dark blue Vajrapani is shown holding a thunderbolt raised over his head in an outstretched hand. The face of the protector is terrible to behold. Yet at the instant that the bit of negative energy that threatens the devout is neutralized, the visage turns to one of tender mercy, showing that Vajrapani is ready to initiate the seeker into the higher spiritual mysteries.

For the Wesak, chant this mantra as you see the Earth's layer of consciousness being cleansed of negative energy.

Mantra Invoking Vajrasattwa, the Being Who Purifies and Protects the Sincere Seeker.

Om Vajra Sattwa Hung

(OM VAHJ-RAH SAHT-WAH HOONG)

Bright bluish white, this Tibetan positive thought-form is used to produce mental clarity. In traditional Tibetan Buddhist meditations, a small, white meditative figure is visualized sitting a foot over one's head. As the mantra is chanted, the figure sends a beam of white light into the top of your head. Subsequently, all manner of foul mental thoughts and habits are released through the aura, chakras, and subtle body. The gunk is then absorbed into the Earth, which knows how to recycle it into usable energy.

To use this mantra for the planet, chant it as you see the Earth releasing the gunk humanity has created into the consuming energy of sunlight. The energy of sunlight cleanses the aura of the Earth every day. By our conscious efforts, we are quickening and concentrating this process.

Mantra Invoking Kwan Yin.

Namo Kwan Shi Yin Pu Sa

[NAH-MOH KOO-AHN SHEE YIN POO SAH]

Kwan Yin is the Chinese feminine form of Avaloketeshwara. Among the Buddhist archetypes, Kwan Yin is a source of great compassion. The consciousness may expand, the knowledge grow, and spiritual abilities manifest, but without compassion these are little better than dust or straw. Jesus indicated this when he told us that without love we have nothing. It is the same idea here. The Kwan Yin mantra infuses the consciousness envelope surrounding the Earth with dynamic compassion, which manifests as grace and mercy. Chant the Kwan Yin mantra and know that you are contributing to the growth of dynamic compassion everywhere.

Mantra Invoking Kalachakra, the Tibetan Shiva.

Om Ha Ksa Ma La Va Ra Yam Swaha

(OM HAH KSAH MAH LAH VAH RAH YAHM SWAH-HA)

Kalachakra is the spirit of the Wheel of Time, the last teaching of the Buddha before his death. Chanting this mantra in a personal way will help you evolve more quickly. Chanting it for the planet will help the Earth on her own spiritual journey.

Shiva, the Siddha Mantra, Leading One on the Path of the Perfected Being.

Om Nama Shivaya

(OM NAH-MAH SHEE-VAH-YAH)

Jesus said, "Be ye perfect, even as your Father in Heaven is perfect." Far Eastern practices of the siddha tradition have taken this dictum seriously centuries before Jesus was born. A siddha is a perfected being. "Perfected" means that the chakras have become perfect in mastering the basic energy principle primarily associated with that chakra. For the base of the spine, the principle is earth; for the second, water; for the third, fire; and so forth.

When Jesus walked upon the water, he demonstrated mastery over the principle governing the second chakra. Moses did the same when he parted the waters for the faithful leaving Egypt. When Jesus calmed the winds upon the sea, he showed his mastery of the fourth chakra. Similarly, when he said, "Heaven and Earth may pass away, but my words shall not pass away," he showed fifth-chakra mastery.

The siddha teachers of India would call Jesus a siddha. One of their principal mantras is *Om Nama Shivaya*. Chant this Hindu mantra with the idea in your mind that all of us should become perfect, each in his or her own way.

Mantra Invoking Saraswati.

Om Eim Saraswatyei Swaha

(OM I'M SAH-RAH-SWAH-TEE-YEA SWAH-HAH)

Saraswati, by whose power of speech (Vach) the universe was created, bestows knowledge of all kinds. Chant the Saraswati mantra with the intention of consciously moving the level of spiritual understanding among humanity to ever-higher levels. Eventually, when we know enough, our bad habits as a species will simply melt away.

Mantra of Avalokiteshwara, Source of the Bodhisattva Vow.

Om Mani Padme Hum

(OM MAH-NEE PAHD-MEY HOOM)

This is the great mantra often translated as: "The jewel of consciousness is in the heart's lotus."

Avaloketeshwara is recorded as a spiritual being who reached such a high level of spiritual attainment that it was as if he had climbed the highest hill and then reached a stone fence at the top of that hill. Once he reached this place, Avaloketeshwara leaped up onto the stone fence and was about to jump over, after which he would enter a new stage of being altogether and pass forever from humankind. At that moment he heard a great moan from behind him. Turning around, he beheld the collective unconscious of humanity beginning to grieve for the loss of his presence. Overcome with compassion, he decided to put off this final stage of enlightenment, his final beatification, for the sake of sentient beings everywhere. That decision became the Boddhisattva Vow, the vow of service to conscious life everywhere. Many serious Buddhists today take that vow. The depth of seriousness of those who take the vow varies, but if you think about it, every great spiritual teacher of mankind must have taken a vow or made a decision similar to this, else why would they come back to help us?

Spiritual discipline using the great *Mani* mantra is done to promote the idea of spiritual advancement combined with service to all sentient life. For the Wesak, chant it knowing that you are putting your metaphysical shoulder to the same wheel the masters and Great Ones are constantly pushing—the wheel of humanity's spiritual advancement.

The Word Has Spread

Since that day in May 1975 when I first started performing the Wesak ceremony, many hundreds of people have attended. At that time it was only I and the Buddhist organizations, as far as I know, that observed the day in a special way for all the work done for us by the followers of the Great Ones. But I am happy to report that Wesak is now widely observed by many different organizations. Though the manner of observation may vary, what we all have in common is a dedication to the achievement of the common spiritual destiny of mankind. I see that destiny as unity born of Love, when hatred and prejudice, violence and ignorance are finally overcome.

If you are so inclined, organize your own Wesak celebration. It does not have to be large or elaborate. It is written in Eastern scripture that God knows the sentiment of the heart, even when the means are slender. If you do just one Wesak observance, even out of curiosity, you will have performed a service for us all. I, for one, will be grateful.

13

Gayatri Mantra: The Essence of All Mantras

Among all the millions of mantras written down and stored in Far Eastern archives, the Gayatri mantra is universally considered the essence of all mantras. The Sanskrit words contain the essential vibration of the upper luminous spheres of light, and all spiritual powers and potencies are within.

According to Vedic cosmology, there are seven luminous spheres of light. Each successive sphere or realm is much more spiritually advanced and sublime than the previous one. In striking resemblance to Paradise in Dante's *The Divine Comedy*, these luminous spheres are progressively attainable through human spiritual development until, finally, we merge with God. We may then return to Earth only if God wishes or needs us to perform some service in the grand scheme of things.

These various realms of light are the abode of saints and sages, prophets and rishis, angels and archangels, and the Great Saviors among humanity who have come from time to time. Although more than one way exists to attain these various realms, a way common to all is the venerable Gayatri mantra.

The Gayatri mantra is simply meditation on spiritual light. While other mantras are great for their purposes, this one is specifically for the purpose of enlightening the mind and intellect. For pure spiritual potency, the accumulation of the highest spiritual light, and attainment of enlightenment, there is nothing to compare with the Gayatri mantra.

Whether practiced by Hindus or Buddhists of diverse kinds, the Gayatri mantra is recognized as supreme in bestowing enlightenment.

According to Vedic teachings, each of the seven luminous spheres
has one single vibration, which is an encapsulated vibration of the entire realm. It is a summary of the sphere in the form of a single word.
When we intone the vibration of that sphere, we bring the vibration
into ourselves. A connection is then created between us and that
realm. At first, the connection is tenuous and faint. But over time,
through sustained spiritual practice, the connection becomes so powerful that one can maintain the vibration of these realms even while in-
habiting physical form during the activities of daily life. In Sanskrit
this state is sometimes called *sahaja samadhi*, or "the natural enlightened state."

Various Far Eastern religious writings contain references to the
seven spheres as well. The Buddhist bodhisattvas have detailed the
realms and qualities of light: "the clear light," "the first bright light,"
and so forth. The Hindu yogis of the Siddha Path (the Path of the Perfected Beings) also guardedly refer to them. Paramahansa Muktananda, world-renowned teacher of the Siddha Path, even wrote
about his "journeys" in his autobiography. Jesus taught, "In my Father's
house are many mansions." Through whatever door we may enter, access to the realms of light is part of our spiritual destiny on Earth, both
individually and as a species. We have the words of the Great Ones as
testimony.

Our Earth is the lowest location among the seven luminous
spheres of light. The vibrational sound for the Earth plane is *Bhuh*. In
some spiritual texts you will find references to the Earth plane as Bhuh
Loka. It should be noted that there are also seven lower, nether (dark)
spheres as well ("as above, so below"). Naturally, many beings from the
lower spheres attempt to reach the first sphere of light, just as we are
trying to reach the higher realms. When beings from the lower spheres
manage to make it here to Earth, havoc ensues. The Vedic scriptures
provide detailed explanations of the interworking between the inhabi-

tants of the realms of light and darkness, but in everyday thought it is the ongoing struggle between good and evil.

The Gayatri mantra uses sound to invoke the vibration of each of the seven luminous layers of the universe specifically into the Earth plane. Furthermore, through repetition of this mantra these vibrations of pure light are invoked directly into us. Prolonged use of the Gayatri mantra will eventually accumulate so much spiritual light in the physical body that it resists decay, even after death.

When the great yogi Paramahansa Yogananda passed from earthly life in 1952, his body was placed in an open coffin where he lay plainly visible for mourners and passersby for twenty-eight days without any observable decay whatsoever. Finally, a small spot of decay appeared on his nose and the coffin was sealed. The event was recorded and reported by *Time* magazine.

Yogananda's organization, the Self-Realization Fellowship, teaches a specific technique for spiritual development. The Gayatri mantra is not that technique. However, Yogananda practiced the Gayatri mantra in his youth, as all Brahmins do. Indeed, in the very earliest editions of *Autobiography of a Yogi*, there is a photograph of him performing a Gayatri fire ceremony for a few assembled students, devotees, and friends. This photo was removed from the book long ago, but those of you who happen to have a very early edition will find it there.

One day in 1984, when I was shopping in Hollywood, California, I chanced upon the SRF gift store. There I met Sister Sita, a sweet, elderly woman who joined the organization as a young girl and became an SRF renunciate while Yogananda was still in the body. On that day, and others which followed, she told me that Yogananda used to perform Gayatri fire ceremonies for the benefit of his students in the early days.

I have practiced the Gayatri mantra since 1974 and I consider it one of the foundations for my spiritual practice. I cannot recommend it highly enough. The prana becomes energized. The light in the aura becomes brighter and brighter. A beneficial energy comes through you that is helpful to everyone. Attunement to the masters who have gone before who have also practiced this mantra grows. An ineffable quiet begins to permeate the mind. I will cease my praise, but not before I tell of two small incidents that taught me its value very early in my practice.

I had been practicing the mantra for only a few short weeks, certainly not long enough to develop any spiritual proficiency. On a trip to Philadelphia from Washington, D.C., I stayed at an urban ashram of spiritual people who also practiced this mantra. The first night after dinner, the director of the household was preparing to wash the dinner dishes and she passed by me very closely on her way to the sink. As she passed, I "heard" silent words coming from the base of her spine. I heard *Om Bhuh . . . Om Bhuh . . . Om Bhuvaha . . . Om Bhuvaha . . . ,* over and over again. This surreal experience went on for about two minutes, then she was called out of the room and the experience was over. It was exceedingly strange. After reflecting upon it, I concluded that I was "hearing" her spiritual discipline. That brief moment is still vividly in my mind all these years later.

Another, more telling incident happened while I was serving as a priest-in-residence for a small Far Eastern–based center in Washington, D.C. During my tenure there, I practiced the Gayatri mantra intensely. My minimum number of repetitions was one thousand a day. Most days I would do more. One day after I had been practicing for three or four years, a visitor rang the bell. This was not an unusual occurrence, but the person ringing the bell was not usual. It was a young Buddhist monk from the Buddhist Vihara (public center) up the street. He was no more than thirty-five years old and had a flashing and infectious grin.

Following spiritual protocol and common courtesy, I invited him in and offered him a cup of tea. I put the water on to boil while I took him on a tour of the small quarters we occupied. After a few minutes, he looked at me intently and remarked, "I see you also do the mystic formula." I said I had no idea what he was talking about. He smiled and began to chant the Gayatri mantra. When my eyebrows went up about a foot, he laughed in a friendly fashion. After a cup of tea and pleasant conversation during which he clearly indicated to me that we shared a common spiritual practice, he went his way.

People with advanced spiritual sight can discern the various qualities of spiritual light invoked by certain mantras. By "seeing" the kind of light in my aura, the young monk was able to tell what mantra I was doing.

Vishwamitra and the Gayatri Mantra

The Gayatri mantra is thousands and thousands of years old. It was first "discovered" and promulgated by a rishi called Vishwamitra, a king who went through many arduous struggles to attain spiritual power. In the beginning Vishwamitra was motivated by envy. But envy was merely a stepping stone to his eventual attainment of more than he ever dreamed possible. There is a great lesson in that one simple idea. Even our most negative and vile qualities can serve as a motivating force for attainment of the higher purposes of life. Here, in brief, is the story that has been told about him for generations.

Vishwamitra was a king in every sense of the word. He had a geographical area in which he was the ruler supreme. He had both loyal subjects and detractors. He tried to take care of the people in the kingdom, but as in every government, there were problems. Sometimes when weather conditions were not favorable, the crops were meager and food for people would run short. At such times he fretted about how to discharge his kingly duties for the benefit of the people. At his core, he was a thoroughly honorable man. While he was not without weaknesses, his intentions as a ruler were sincere.

It was just after a skimpy harvest that Vishwamitra took his entourage to the forest for a few days of hunting and reflection. Near the evening of the first day, he and his band of soldiers and attendants came upon the hermitage of a rishi. As it turned out, Vishwamitra had

stumbled upon the forest retreat of the powerful and famous Brahma-
rishi Vasistha. The title Brahma-rishi indicates a sage of the highest order. One who attains this state stands at the pinnacle of knowledge
possible to attain while occupying a human form.

When Vishwamitra and his party approached the modest hut
where Vasistha usually meditated, the rishi came out and greeted the
king warmly. He offered food to the king and his men. Vishwamitra
was courteous and genuinely concerned for the welfare of the great
sage. Out of consideration for the rishi, the king said that he and his
men were many and that the rishi should not deplete his food supplies,
particularly during a time when harvests had been poor.

Vasistha replied that this would not be a problem. He went behind
his hut and returned leading a haltered cow. He then said to the cow,
"Provide a table of plenty for the king and his men." Immediately there
appeared an ample repast spread upon cloths on the ground. There
was enough to feed everyone easily. The king was stunned. They all sat
to eat, and the rishi bade the king to sit next to him.

Once seated and eating, the king told Vasistha about the troubles
of running his kingdom, with all of its problems, and wryly observed
that one of the problems was unpredictable crop yields that made it
difficult to feed the people.

In the back of his mind, King Vishwamitra was hatching a plan
that grew more detailed every moment. As they spoke he carefully laid
the groundwork and began to move toward his main objective. Since
the year had provided a slim harvest for the kingdom, the king suggested to Brahma-rishi Vasistha that the cow-that-produced-anything
could better serve humanity if it were in the king's possession. After
subtly building a case upon "the good of the people," the king asked
Vasistha to give him the cow.

The sage nodded his head and acknowledged that what the king
said was noble and true. It would serve the kingdom well if the king had
such a cow. But, the sage said quite firmly, he could not give Vishwamitra the cow. Such a magical animal was the sole spiritual province

of a Brahma-rishi. Brahma-rishi Vasistha apologized for not being able to meet the king's request and continued eating.

King Vishwamitra would not be dissuaded and upped the ante. Conditions of want, hinted the king, demanded aggressive measures to combat the enemy of the people: hunger. Extreme conditions very likely could generate some "emergency mandate" whereby he could confiscate the cow for the general good. Vasistha merely grunted.

When there was no further response from the Brahma-rishi, the king ordered his soldiers to go and take the cow by its leash. But as the soldiers attempted to seize the animal, Vasistha said a few Sanskrit words to the cow and it moved rapidly away. The soldiers followed, trying unsuccessfully to grab the leash. Each time the soldiers approached, the cow eluded them. Finally the king became agitated. If the sage would not comply, the king said, he would be taken prisoner. Again, Vasistha merely grunted. When the king's men rushed the sage and tried to capture him, they had no better success than when they had tried to capture the cow. Every time they got close, the sage would mysteriously disappear, only to reappear in another location. (This is reminiscent of Jesus hiding himself from the masses. In almost every religious tradition the advanced ones demonstrate miraculous powers.)

Finally the king lost all patience. He was not accustomed to being refused in any matter. Impulsively, he threatened to have his bowmen shoot the sage. Vasistha grunted, unperturbed. Having committed himself, the king now had no choice. By his own words he was forced to act, even if it was only to save face. He lined up the bowmen and they loosed their arrows at Vasistha. But as the arrows approached him, the Brahma-rishi merely lowered his staff and all the arrows entered it and were swallowed up in an instant. Looking at Vishwamitra he said, "Shall I swallow up your bowmen also?"

The king was now genuinely furious, but he was smart enough to know when he was beaten. He gathered up his men and their belongings, and they all returned to the palace. However, he was preoccupied with Vasistha and haunted by the idea of the cow with miraculous abilities. He could not get it out of his head. He fumed to himself that Vasistha was duty bound to give him the cow. Yet the sage had refused. Vishwamitra convinced himself that Vasistha was disloyal and did not have the good of the people at heart. The king thought all of this and more. But mostly he knew, deep inside, that he was envious of the sage.

The sage had power. Real power. And although the king had position and prestige, he did not have real power. Not the kind that mattered. As his inner denunciation of the sage grew more and more acrid, his envy also grew. Finally, overcome by his own envy, he made a decision. He would develop the same kind of power within himself and he would beat Vasistha at his own game.

So thinking, Vishwamitra left his kingdom. He renounced his position, title, and possessions and retreated into the mountains, where he began an austere program of meditation and concentration designed to bring all manner of powers to his mind. He was determined to prevail and take that cow by force, if necessary. And if he humiliated Brahmarishi Vasistha in the bargain, so much the better. With an adamantine resolve, he dove deeper and deeper into meditation.

After several years, the power of his decision and the strength of his discipline were such that the celestials in a higher spiritual realm noticed Vishwamitra's efforts. Indra, chief of the celestials, became concerned. With such resolve and inner drive, thought Indra, Vishwamitra might eventually try to supplant him. So Indra decided to try some diversionary tactics. He went to recruit a certain dazzlingly beautiful celestial woman he knew who always liked a good challenge.

One day, as Vishwamitra was deep in his spiritual practices, he heard a strange sound like the jingling of tiny bells. After hearing them for some time, he could no longer restrain his curiosity, so he opened one eye to see if he could spy the source of the sound. He was completely unprepared for what greeted his eye. There before him was an exquisitely beautiful woman. She wore a sari of many colors draped artfully over her curvaceous form. And she was dancing. How wonderfully she was dancing!

Vishwamitra opened his other eye and the woman smiled. The radiance of her smile stirred him deep within his loins, and Vishwamitra found that his desire to meditate was diminishing with every moment. *Ching ting-ting. Ching ting-ting.* The woman danced enchantingly to the chime of her hand cymbals. Soon Vishwamitra was completely entranced. The woman came over and sat down beside him. "What is your name, O handsome and powerful one?" she asked. That did it. He became totally enamored of her in the space of time between two seconds, and completely forgot about his meditations, the sage Vasistha, the wish-fulfilling cow, and everything but this wonderful new companion.

Over the next two years, Vishwamitra and the celestial nymph, Menaka, made love and dallied by mountain streams. It was truly idyllic. And Indra was pleased, for it was he who had recruited Menaka to go to Vishwamitra and take his mind off his spiritual practices. Although Vishwamitra was very happy for a time, one day the memory of his meditations returned to him. So he said to Menaka, "I think I will go and meditate for a while."

Immediately Menaka flew into a rage and told him that if he did that, she would just leave and he would be completely alone again.

Vishwamitra was stunned. This was not the woman he had thought he knew for the last two years. He tried to reason with her about his meditations, explaining that he would be gone for only a couple of hours, but she would have none of it. Finally he grew suspicious and asked the questions he had never asked before. Where had she come from, anyway? How did she find him in his high mountain retreat? Had she been looking for him? As his suspicion grew, Menaka saw that she could not influence him, and she disappeared in a cloud of blue smoke. Shocked, Vishwamitra sat down on a rock and collected his thoughts. How had this happened? Who was she? What had he been doing, and how, suddenly, had he lost two years of time?

He realized that he had entirely forgotten about his desire to attain a high spiritual state. Any thoughts of besting Brahma-rishi Vasistha had vanished. Now those thoughts came rushing back and flooded him anew with a desire to meditate. With a firm resolve, he climbed to a spot a thousand feet farther up the slopes and began his spiritual discipline anew.

He had lost most of his spiritual advancement. His concentration had slipped, and his mind wandered without control from this memory to that idea with no logical sequence or reasonable intent, as if his mind belonged to no one. But he was determined to gain control over his thoughts once again. He was entirely resolved that his mind would conform to his will, and not the other way around.

After several years of concentrated meditative pursuits, Vishwamitra surpassed his previous state. His concentration became firm and his mind could contemplate any subject with a continuous stream of mental investigation. He was breaking new ground in his meditation practices.

Indra again became concerned for his status as chief of the celestials. Assuming that what had worked once would work again, he sent another celestial woman to tempt Vishwamitra out of his meditation. This time, however, when Vishwamitra heard the *ching ting-ting, ching ting-ting* of the finger cymbals, his attention never wavered. With a steely inner focus, he kept on with his discipline. But the celestial woman came closer and closer, her finger cymbals became louder and louder, and her perfume caressed his nostrils. Vishwamitra became irritated. In a moment's flash of anger, he sent out a measure of his considerable spiritual power and turned her into a rock, consuming in this single act a huge amount of his spiritual attainment. Immediately, Vishwamitra found that his powers of understanding had diminished. The translucent understanding of existence that had been the object of his meditations slipped away. What he had formerly understood was gone from his mind. He now groped for a key to his former knowledge. He had slid back down from the heights he had attained. (As for the woman, the avatar Rama would appear many years later and restore her human form, and then send her to a high spiritual state.)

Vishwamitra was disappointed and disgusted with himself, but undaunted. He climbed another five hundred feet up the mountain, found a new spot, and once more immersed himself in meditation. He was still determined to reach a state of development superior to that of Brahma-rishi Vasistha.

Meanwhile, in a nearby part of the country, a king named Trishanku was getting old. As rulers go, King Trishanku had been very good. He had led a good life, ruled for the people's welfare, and was well regarded for his astute management of the affairs of state. Since death was fast approaching, he desired to ascend into heaven in his physical body. Knowing that Brahma-rishi Vasistha was close by, he sent a messenger to him and asked the sage to come to his court. When the two of them were alone, the king told the sage of his desire to ascend into heaven in his physical body. Vasistha lowered his gaze and shook his head. "It would be contrary to Divine Law. I cannot do this for you. Please ask for something else." The king wanted nothing else and the two parted company.

After Vasistha had left, a wandering mendicant brought the king news of a powerful new sage meditating in the Himalayas. King Trishanku requested the mendicant to go ask that powerful sage to perform the fire ceremony that would allow him to ascend into heaven in his physical body.

Vishwamitra was deep in meditation when the mendicant approached him. He stirred not even one eyelash. He was rock still and deep in a divine meditative embrace. Knowing that even in such a high state Vishwamitra could hear him, the man joined his palms and made the request on behalf of the king. Vishwamitra made no response. At last, the mendicant noted that the great sage Brahma-rishi Vasistha had been unable to perform the ceremony. That did it. It was an irresistible opportunity. "Who knows when such a chance will come my way again?" Vishwamitra thought. Vishwamitra immediately came out of meditation and smiled broadly. "I shall do it. I shall help King Trishanku attain heaven while still in his physical body."

It was only a day's journey to King Trishanku's palace, and the road was well traveled. Vishwamitra and the mendicant made the trip easily. Upon arrival, they were greeted with celebration as important dignitaries. Vishwamitra enjoyed this show of respect and his anticipation grew for the day when he would show up Brahma-rishi Vasistha. He immediately began making plans for a huge fire ceremony during which he would send the king to heaven in his physical form.

Two days later the ceremony began. It was to last three days. After the first day, crowds from the neighboring provinces swelled to several hundred. After the second day a thousand people had shown up to see the king ascend while still in his physical form. On the third day, Vishwamitra began the rites that would accomplish the feat. After several hours, the king arose from his seat and began to ascend into the evening sky. Up, up, up, he went. Higher and higher into the deepening dark of night. Soon he was nearly out of sight. But just as he was about to be lost from view, the king was spotted by Indra.

Quoting the spiritual law that no one may travel into the higher realms of light while in a physical form, Indra sent the king plunging headfirst back to Earth. The powerful words uttered by Indra were backed by spiritual law. As Vishwamitra watched, horrified, his mind raced. What should he do now? Over a thousand people were watching at this very moment. King Trishanku raced toward the ground, crying out to Vishwamitra for help. If the king crashed into Earth, Vishwamitra would be humiliated forever. He had to think of something, and fast.

In a flash it came to him. Putting forth his hand, he used his spiritual force, and with a thundering command he ordered the king's body to stop its movement. The power of his spiritual discipline gave authority to his words. The king's body came to an abrupt stop in midflight, and there he stayed. He could not rise because it would violate Divine Law. He could not fall because of the power of Vishwamitra's command. By a divine compromise that satisfied spiritual law, a new constellation was named in honor of the king. There in the East, to this day, a group of stars shows Trishanku standing upside down in the night sky.

Though he had escaped disaster, Vishwamitra was chagrined. Once again he had used a portion of his spiritual attainments to satisfy a passing desire. He wondered if he would ever grow wise. But his spirit was indomitable. Again he climbed the mountain to perform his spiritual disciplines. For a long time he practiced secret and powerful mantra formulas and performed pranayama, spiritually scientific deep breathing (described in chapter 7). He lived on snow and air alone. Deeper and deeper he went into meditation.

Finally, Vishwamitra's profound efforts came to the attention of Brahma, the Creator. Brahma was impressed with the indefatigable efforts of the sage who had been a king, and he appeared to Vishwamitra and blessed him. He gave him the title of Maha-rishi, or "great sage." He further instructed Vishwamitra that if he wanted to be a Brahma-rishi, he must go seek the blessing of Brahma-rishi Vasistha.

Vishwamitra was incensed. That Vasistha guy again? He had done years and years of spiritual discipline, only to have the name of that sage thrown in his face—and by none other than Brahma himself! Vishwamitra became cold with resolve. Something decisive must be done.

When Vishwamitra arrived at the Brahma-rishi's hut, Vasistha and his wife, Arundhati, who shared his high state of consciousness, were having a conversation. Vishwamitra could not quite make out what they were saying, but he decided to be ready with a deadly plan if Brahma-rishi Vasistha should emerge from the hut. Glancing around, he noticed a large rock and concluded that it would be perfect to smash Vasistha's head with when he emerged from the doorway. So thinking, he picked up the rock, crept over to the doorway, and raised the rock over his head. He could now hear the conversation going on inside.

Arundhati was speaking to her husband. "He has become so great! It is only fitting and proper that you bless him."

Vasistha replied, "I will. I intend to give him the highest blessing."

Vishwamitra wondered who they were talking about.

Arundhati continued. "You are going to make him a Brahma-rishi?"

Vasistha vigorously replied, "Absolutely! He has passed every test.

Vishwamitra has proved himself worthy in every way. No matter what the difficulty, he has persevered. He was originally motivated by envy, anger, and revenge. Then he overcame the better part of those negative qualities. He was sidetracked by lust, but he saw his mistake and once again returned to his meditation practices. He was seduced by ego-bound ambition to show me up with King Trishanku. But still he returned and persevered. His spirit has become so steeped in the divine vibrations that even Brahma has blessed him. He is thoroughly prepared for the highest state of enlightenment. All he has to do is come to my feet and I will joyfully bestow the title, rank, and state of Brahma-rishi upon him."

Vishwamitra heard these words and his heart melted. He felt such a shame that he could hardly bear it. He reflected upon all of his negative qualities and understood in a rush that Brahma-rishi Vasistha had been rooting for him all along to attain the higher states available to the ardent seeker of truth. He now thoroughly understood that only the sublime understanding of a Brahma-rishi could possess and rightfully manage the power to fulfill any desire at will, such as Vasistha had demonstrated with the cow. The responsibility of such an ability is enormous. It was now obvious why Vasistha had refused him the cow. The idea of his having it in his previous low state was absurd. It would have been spiritually irresponsible for Vasistha to have given him the cow.

In disgust at his own arrogance and foolishness, Vishwamitra began to beat his own head with the rock. Inside, the divine couple could hear the *thump, thump, thump* of the rock as it crashed into Vishwamitra's head by his own hand. They rushed outside to see what was causing this odd noise.

Seeing Vishwamitra's bloody head, Vasistha ran up and stayed the hand with the rock. "Here! Stop! What are you doing?" Vishwamitra burst into tears and begged for forgiveness for his faults and evil intention. He collapsed in a heap at the feet of Brahma-rishi Vasistha. A great divine current sprang from the feet of Vasistha and coursed through Vishwamitra's body. Every cell in his body was bathed in that powerful current. The hair all over his body stood on end. Tears of devotion sprang from his eyes. In just a few seconds, he was completely transformed.

Vishwamitra went into spontaneous samadhi, or divine communion. He sat up, wrapped in an indescribable bliss, at one with the entire universe. Deep in that reverie, he heard mystical sounds: *Om Bhuh . . . Om Bhuvaha . . . Om Swaha . . . Om Maha . . . Om Janaha . . . Om Tapaha . . . Om Satyam . . . Om Tat Satvitur Varenyam . . . Bhargo Devasya Dhimahi . . . Dhiyo Yonaha Prachodayat.* He was hearing the sounds of the vibration of the seven great upper luminous levels of creation itself.

The Supreme had given to Vishwamitra the gift of Gayatri mantra, the mantra of the universe itself in all its upper spheres of spiritual light.

Vishwamitra had become the seer of the Gayatri mantra. He was the first to realize the essence of the luminous spheres through single, powerful vibrations that contain the essence of each realm. He was the first to bring to Earth a gift that would free many millennia of earnest seekers through a discipline employing but a single mantra. And these thousands of years later, the mantra is still practiced and great attainments are still made using it. In practicing this mantra, part of the opening prayer should be a brief salutation to Brahma-rishi Vishwamitra and his guru, Brahma-rishi Vasistha. Without Brahma-rishi Vishwamitra's travails, we might not have that mantra here on Earth today. Without the grace of Brahma-rishi Vasistha, Vishwamitra might not have become the seer of this great mantra. Here is the Gayatri mantra.

Gayatri Mantra:
Long and Short Forms

There are two renditions of the Gayatri mantra. They are referred to simply as the long form and the short form.

Long Form.

Om Bhuh, Om Bhuvaha, Om Swaha
Om Maha, Om Janaha, Om Tapaha,
Om Satyam Om Tat Savitur Varenyam
Bhargo Devasya Dhimahi
Dhiyo Yonaha Prachodayat

(OM BOO OM BOO-VAH-HA OM SWAH-HA

OM MAH-HA OM JAH-NAH-HA OM TAH-PAH-HA

OM-SAHT-YAHM OM TAHT SAH-VEE-TOOR VAHR-EHN-YUM

BHAHR-GO DEH-VAHS-YAH DEE-MAH-HEE

DEE-YOH YOHN-AH-HA PRAH-CHOH-DAH-YAHT)

*"O Self-effulgent Light that has given birth to all the lokas
[spheres of consciousness], who is worthy of worship and appears
through the orbit of the Sun, illumine our intellect."*

Here is a list of the spiritual planes represented (encapsulated) in
the Gayatri mantra.

Om Bhuh (first chakra)	Earth plane
Om Bhuvaha (second chakra)	Atmospheric plane
Om Swaha (third chakra)	Solar region
Om Maha (fourth chakra)	First spiritual region beyond the Sun: heart vibration
Om Janaha (fifth chakra)	Second spiritual region beyond the Sun: power of the divine spiritual Word
Om Tapaha (sixth chakra)	Third spiritual region beyond the Sun: sphere of the Progenitors; realm of the highest spiritual understanding while still identified with existence as an individual being

Om Satyam (seventh chakra)	Abode of supreme Truth: absorption into the Supreme
Om Tat Savitur Varenyam	That realm of Truth which is beyond human comprehension
Bhargo Devasya Dhimahi	In that place where all the celestials of all the
Dhiyo Yonaha Prachodayat	spheres have received enlightenment, kindly enlighten our intellect

There are several useful things to observe about the structure of the mantra. First, notice that the syllable *Om* is used as a prefix to all of the mystical words that represent the realms. There is good reason for this. While on Earth, we work with our conscious attention focused through the will. Our will is expressed in our daily decisions and behavior. The biospiritual location of our will is centered at the brow center, a point that is between the eyebrows and raised a few centimeters. In normal waking life, our eyes are very close to this center of will. When we close our eyes to meditate, this is the place where our gaze should be focused. The seed spiritual sound for this place is *Om*.

If we are engaged in a spiritual discipline to bring the spiritual essence of the various realms of light into the physical world, we need to do this with consciousness and will. This is accomplished by using *Om* as a prefix to the sounds of those individual realms of light. This also means that we enjoy interaction with all the realms through self-awareness and intentional activity.

When we reach the phrase that begins *Bhargo Devasya*, we are performing a spiritual invocation that includes every being who has ever become enlightened or who has used this particular mantra. We are entreating the consciously manifesting forces of the universe to assist us in our cause of achieving enlightenment. There are stages of enlightenment that are represented by the individual realms. Now we are asking for help in attaining the supreme goal of the species.

Short Form.

Om Bhuh, Bhuvaha, Swaha
Om Tat Savitur Varenyam
Bhargo Devasya Dhimahi
Dhiyo Yonaha Prachodayat

(OM BOO BOO-VAH-HAH SWAH-HA

OM TAHT SAH-VEE-TOOR VAHR-EHN-YUM

BHAHR-GO DEH-VAHS-YAH DEE-MAH-HEE

DEE-YOH YOHN-AH-HA PRAH-CHOH-DAH-YAHT)

*"O Self-effulgent Light that has given birth to all the lokas
[spheres of consciousness], who is worthy of worship and appears
through the orbit of the Sun, illumine our intellect."*

For reasons I do not understand, the short form of the mantra is much more commonly practiced in the Far East than the long form. I have repeatedly asked Eastern spiritual teachers why this is so, but I have never received a satisfactory answer.

Which Form Is Best to Use?

When I was initiated into the practice of the Gayatri mantra, the form I was given was the long form. I did not even know that a short form existed. For that reason, I did not ask my initiator what the difference was between the two. Never having received much of an answer from any other teacher, I can recommend the long form based only upon my experience with it.

Earlier I spoke of the benefits of this mantra. I will add a bit more here. I have shared this mantra with a handful of earnest seekers over the years. Without exception they reported back to me that new levels of peace descended into their minds after just a few days of practice. Some reported that they began to fathom things about their lives which had eluded their previous understanding. They universally expressed gratitude for receiving the mantra, viewing it as a true spiritual gift. I can only add to those expressions my own gratitude to Brahma-rishi Vasistha, Brahma-rishi Vishwamitra, and my spiritual initiator, without whose collective beneficence I would not have written this work.

Finally, each of us who attains higher levels of spiritual development while living on Earth performs a service for the planet and her inhabitants. Humanity has a destiny shepherded by the Great Ones. We individually may choose to share in the work toward that destiny. As such choices are made, it becomes easier for humanity as a whole to advance. As such choices are made over the centuries, one day all of humanity will reach a spiritual critical mass and be changed forever. The Gayatri mantra plays an important God-given role in the uplifting of the entire species. So whether your goals are personal or altruistic, this mantra can be of great benefit.

14

Teachers and Gurus

During the last thirty years there has been a steady influx of spiritual leaders and teachers from the Far East. Instructed by them, Americans have adopted the idea of the guru or enlightened spiritual teacher who guides the faithful on the path to enlightenment, self-realization, or communion with the divine beloved. The teacher, it is taught, assumes responsibility for the development of the student. Correspondingly, the more the student follows the leadership of the teacher, the faster the progress of the student. This is the overall idea of the guru-disciple relationship.

Contrary to what many spiritual teachers have told us, the guru is not a person but a principle. If a large generator sits quietly without distributing power, it nonetheless contains power within. Just because the power is not operating does not mean it is not there, nor that it will not suddenly turn on if the need arises. Similarly, the guru exists in each of us as a principle that may or may not be operating at any given moment. At various times in various lifetimes according to our soul's own blueprint, the guru principle begins to operate. The true guru is not some person to whom you give complete and slavish obedience. The true guru is a principle that resides in your own heart and will lead you, as you are ready, on your spiritual journey of many winding paths. In Sanskrit, this guru principle is called the *upaguru*, or "teacher without form."

The syllables *gu* and *ru* mean "darkness" and "that which dispels it." The guru is that which dispels the darkness of ignorance. Since the soul, or atman, is always in a state of light and enlightenment, then that which is in darkness is our mind. The mind does not know the true nature of the soul without some help. To bring the mind to an understanding that it must seek the light, find the light, and ultimately surrender to the light is the function of the guru principle. Enlightenment means an enlightened mind.

Teachers who have made substantial progress in transforming themselves into oneness with the light, or surrendered themselves in service to it in some way, are "gurus" in common parlance. That is, they are farther along on our common journey and they offer a helping hand. So far so good.

For some teachers, however, subtle changes in their "help" begin to appear. They may demand unquestioning obedience. They may construct fanciful circumstances for us to navigate to "test" us. They may instill not just respect but fear in their students. Somewhere in this scenario, the teacher can cease being a spiritual aid and actually become a hindrance.

There are now and always have been well-qualified, well-intentioned, and beneficial spiritual teachers in almost every religious path. Nothing written here should be construed to mean that teachers are not a good thing or even necessary in some situations or for some people. They are both of these things. But they are also human. And human beings are not perfect. They are capable of error and they have desires just like the rest of us. The main point to keep in the forefront of your mind is that any external teacher is useful to your spiritual progress only so long as he or she presents an accurate reflection of what your inner teacher is trying to show you. The moment the outer teacher does not reflect the inner teacher, then the outer teacher is a hindrance.

All of this runs counter to the well-publicized guru-disciple tradition practiced in both Hinduism and Buddhism. Yet the upaguru principle is well established in their own esoteric texts. The concept has also been recognized in the West, although in a different guise.

Psychologist Carl Jung has contributed the idea of synchronicity to our Western worldview. Synchronicity simply means that unrelated phenomena may have a seeming causal relationship to the observer. For example, you suddenly start thinking of a person who has been close to you but you have not seen for some time because a song related to your memory of the person starts playing on the radio. Then miraculously, within a few seconds, the telephone rings and it is that person. Jung called this a synchronous event. The teachings of the Far East call this the workings of the upaguru.

But if the upaguru is so effective, then it would seem that we would never need an outer teacher or guru. We would just follow the inner teacher and all would go well. But sometimes there may be no real way for our mind to know where the inner teacher is leading. At such times, our best path is to seek and follow the guidance of someone who is more advanced.

There are problems associated with this decision, of course. Since we are the lesser advanced, we may not really know who is the more advanced and who is merely somewhat advanced. Nearly all seekers find themselves in this predicament at one time or another in their spiritual development. The way out of this predicament is in spiritual discipline such as mantra.

Our practice of mantra strengthens the conscious link between the mind and the operation of the upaguru principle. If we need to spend time with a teacher, the practice of our own discipline will lead us to the right one. Continued practice will ensure that we stay only as long as we should, be it a day, a year, or ten years. A student may, for spiritual reasons, spend an entire life with a given teacher. But it is much more common for a person to have several teachers during a lifetime, because each soul has its own blueprint for development.

As we practice mantra, benefits and attributes often come to us. The voice may become imbued with a subtle power as the chakras resonate with more and more energy. The chanted mantras themselves grow in power in the person who practices them. At some point after much practice, the power of the mantra reaches a stage where the mere repetition of it has power for anyone within hearing. It is here that one has reached a stage where he or she may "initiate" others in the practice of the mantra, as is done in the guru-disciple tradition.

Initiation in this context means imparting a mantra "with power" to a deserving student. The mantra is given "with power" so that students may advance much more quickly than if they merely practiced the mantra themselves from scratch. The power of initiation from a qualified teacher can cut several years, or several lifetimes, off the endeavors of a student.

This is a great gift. It is for this reason that the guru-disciple relationship has become entrenched in spiritual traditions of the Far East. But even here, the physical teacher or guru is merely an instrument of the upaguru, your own inner guide.

The true spiritual teacher knows that the upaguru is the teacher without form, the teacher within both student and spiritual guide. The true spiritual teacher knows that it is the upaguru that prods us to become seekers after truth in the first place, and that it is the upaguru which leads us to a qualified teacher at some point.

The nature of our spiritual physiology, as discussed in chapter 2, will ensure that the practice of mantra produces significant results. It cannot be otherwise. But the right teacher at the right time can speed our journey to the goal of enlightenment.

So honor the teacher who may come into your life and be grateful for what you receive. But never forget that even the greatest teachers are merely servants of your own inner guru. For if the outer teachers are truly great, they seek only to serve. The truly advanced and knowledgeable spiritual teachers are not attached to their students.

Many of us have had a time come when we knew beyond doubt that it was time to move on from an organization or teacher. It may be that we have met one or more very valuable teachers and stayed for some time. But at some moment, the inner teacher made clear that the time was up and it was now time to go. Or perhaps the teacher died. At some point, we must honor what we have received from a given teacher in a certain place, and follow the upaguru to the next lesson in the next place.

Most of us are responding to the constant urgings of the upaguru. The inner teacher uses the outer world with all its contents as a school for our development. The upaguru may lead us to this minister or that teacher for a while. Then we may find that we change traditions altogether for a time. I have seen people who have wandered from Vedic Hinduism to Buddhism, and then take off for several years in pursuit of Native American wisdom. Then later they appear, following a more orthodox Jewish or Christian path. Not once, but many times have I seen students following some variation of this winding path as they hearken to the urgings of the upaguru. But to whatever form of religious practice people on the mystical path return, they are never the same as when they started.

Almost without exception, the return to an orthodox spiritual path is now cloaked in a universal kind of understanding. Seekers know that God is in every religion, every path. They know that just because one's own siren song leads 180 degrees away from that of one's neighbor, no one has a corner on absolute truth. As Jesus said, "In my Father's house are many mansions. If it were not true, I would have told you."

To ensure that your inner teacher has an unobstructed path to your conscious mind, the mantra below is useful. It is noteworthy that this mantra contains the seed *Gum* that is traditionally connected with Ganesha and the removing of obstacles. This mantra helps remove the obstacles between our own inner guidance and our conscious, wakeful mind.

Om Gum Gurubhyo Namaha

(OM GOOM GOO-ROO-BYO NAHM-AH-HA)

*"Om and salutations to that which removes the darkness
of ignorance and all impediments thereto."*

15

Who Do You Want to Be?

We are born in a specific time and place. Our genetic code is specific and exact. At a casual glance, it seems that an unlimited horizon of possibilities lies open to us in life. We can do anything we want, become anything or anyone we desire. By effort of will and work we can accomplish anything. Or so we think.

When we are born in the universe, our life spreads before us with unimaginable potentialities. But these seemingly unending possibilities are partially an illusion.

The station of our birth, both geographically and culturally, begins to define our choices: Have we been born into wealth and prominence or poverty and want? Our DNA begins to define our choices: Are we to be plain or handsome? Mentally and physically vital and healthy, or weak and ailing?

Then the karma of our astrological blueprint begins to be felt. The qualities of our solar placement begin to influence wants, desires, choices, and predispositions. The planetary alignments present energy patterns of ease or difficulty, influencing not only events but also our personality as we are forced to adapt to the good or bad potentialities contained in the alignments.

Next, the part of karma from the dormant repository of past actions and decisions from previous lifetimes lies waiting to release with inexorably powerful effect when the appropriate circumstance arises.

Almost immediately after we are shown what seem like unlimited possibilities, a number of limiting forces arise.

Unlike plants, conscious volitional life includes the element of choice and decision. This is the great divide between sentience and nonsentience. While we cannot avoid responding to the laws of physics that govern everything in our bodies, from hydrostatic pressure of capillary action to the need for sleep, we cannot help but respond to our karma and to our drive for advancement. These forces drive us individually and as a species. Still, humanity has the power of choice.

We make choices every day. It is the nature of these choices and the consequences that spring from them that determine the many events and occurrences of our lives. Our decisions stitch and dye the fabric of our existence from day to day and life to life.

Esoteric Levers

Consciousness inevitably includes intentional activity. Certain decisions and actions can be likened to levers that act upon our lives. Colloquially, we speak of pulling ourselves up by our own bootstraps. This is a good analogy. Ancient spiritual disciplines invoke powerful spiritual forces that act in many ways.

The actions that mantras can produce can be as gentle and mild as dropping a stone in a placid pool where the ripples go out gently but with far-reaching effects in the local universe of the pond. Or they can be as powerful as blasting with dynamite until the river feeding the pool changes course to flow along an entirely new path with widespread effect.

It all depends upon how intensely we undertake these disciplines and where we were when we started. If we have practiced in other lifetimes, then we may merely be continuing what we have done before. Progress may be rapid. Possibly, we are starting these new disciplines in this life. In that case, progress can be linked to the general state of our karma at the time we started. No one can say for certain.

Any spiritual discipline is a lever for changing things in life. The things we want to change can be small or they can be monumental. Sometimes we think we can tell the difference, when in fact we are quite ignorant of the effects that may be produced by certain actions.

Let us suppose, for instance, that a person desires wealth. Mantra formulas can eventually produce this condition. The time to achieve it depends upon the past karma of the individual, the intensity of discipline, the amount of time dedicated each day to practicing the discipline, the cumulative amount of time dedicated to achieving the goal, and so forth.

Let us further suppose that a person with relatively little understanding of the Law of Karma or karmic consequences of actions finds and practices a mantra discipline that will lead to material wealth. Let us assume that this discipline is practiced powerfully and faithfully until the goal is achieved. Now, a whole new field of potential karmic activity comes into play, bringing new questions. How will wealth affect the decision-making process of the newly prosperous individual? Will this person become tough and calculating to keep and increase the wealth? Will he or she be sensitive to the needs of others and become philanthropic?

It is not possible to know what we will do in the future under all conditions. But it is possible for us to determine what kind of person we want to become, and to strive to become that. For as we strive for particular outcomes along the way, that state of our being will come into play under all circumstances.

This is the ultimate and final goal of all spiritual discipline, including the practice of Sanskrit mantra.

Who Do You Want to Be?

The achievement of virtue and an ideal state of being is the principal goal of spiritual discipline. You may decide you want to be a "good person," a "spiritual person," or a "righteous person."

We can decide that we wish to attain union with one of the great spiritual figures in history. Some people decide that their highest spiritual ideal is to be one with the Body of Christ. Or to be in union with Krishna forever. Or to be an Enlightened One like the Buddha or to be a conscious participant in the ongoing work of the Cosmic Mind, Transcendental Purusha, or Great Oversoul (it goes by many names). Every day, a very few people make these kinds of spiritual decisions. But the effects of these few decisions and the active pursuit of ideals based upon these decisions will determine the very fate of humanity over time.

So as we near the end of our discussion of Sanskrit mantra, begin the important decision-making process of plumbing the heart of your own spiritual nature for your spiritual ideal. Once you have found it, dedicate all of your spiritual practices and disciplines toward the ultimate achievement of your ideal nature and its fulfillment.

This does not mean that you must forego intermediate goals such as wealth, a happy marriage, a good job, good health, or other things. It merely means that you have framed an ultimate destination that is based in your own nature. From there you proceed with the understanding that the road and the destination are really one.

What will you do with wealth? What will you do with real power? What do you want to accomplish, both within and without? For instance, how can you achieve a state of Love other than by loving? The answers to these questions will determine your fate over many lives.

May Your Efforts Be Successful

This volume has been dedicated to helping you solve the material and spiritual problems of life by providing you with the tool of Sanskrit mantra to help change conditions in which you find yourself.

If you are a bit bewildered because this is your first exposure to mantra-based disciplines, yet you desire to undertake some discipline using mantra, try this approach. After reading this book, take a break for a few days. Don't think about mantras at all. But when you go to sleep, ask for guidance concerning what mantra discipline would be best for you. After three days of this activity, pick up this book again. Scan the table of contents and see if any one chapter seems to have more energy for you than other chapters. Consult that chapter. There may well now be a chapter that seems to appeal to you more than the others. There may be a mantra in that chapter which you can use in your present circumstances with great effect. If not, just leaf through the book until something seems to grab your attention for some reason.

Whatever you finally decide to try, may your practice of Sanskrit mantra serve you well and exceed all of your expectations in fulfillment of your material needs and spiritual objectives.

May you become in practice all that you are in potential. May the love that informs every cell in your body permeate every thought in your mind. May the joy of the universe flow through you every moment. And may the power of the Supreme compassionately empower your actions and fulfill your needs. Achieving this, you will know:

Tattwam Asi

(TAHT-WAHM AH-SEE)

"You are that which you seek."
(Literally "I am that.")

Finally, may the energy of Love encompass you completely. If we are healed in all ways, we inevitably arrive at a state of Love.

1. **Love is based upon Unity.** To love something is to be part of it in some way.
2. **Love involves Understanding.** We inevitably know something about the beloved to love it. And the beloved reveals its secrets to the lover.
3. **Love is an expression of Selflessness.** The ego with its desires and petty concerns is subordinated to something else.

4. **Love is Transcendental.** Beyond human limits, Love often evokes miracles that respond to the call of Love alone.

5. **In Love, the means and the ends are one and the same.** There is no way to achieve the condition or state of Love other than by loving.

6. **Love can be a gift from God.**

7. **Love means service.** Love quickly moves from the realm of the expressible into the realm of the inexpressible. We soon run out of ways to express it. Yet avenues of expression through service to others abound.

8. **The search for Love is the end of all meaning.** If we lust after power, yet have no Love, our search will be dry and our attainments hollow.

9. **Love is our birthplace, our final refuge, and our reason for being.** If we recognize that Compassion and Love are the ultimate destination of our search, the Heart of the Universe itself responds.

May you know within your own heart:

Aham Prema

(AH-HAHM PREH-MAH)

"I Am Divine Love."

Glossary of Sanskrit
and Other Terms

Adepts Spiritually advanced beings with esoteric abilities and knowledge.

Aditi The ninth name of the Sun among the twelve names or powers of the Sun.

Ahankara Conceit.

Ajna Chakra Spiritual center between the eyebrows, often referred to as the sixth chakra, where the masculine and feminine currents in the body meet and join. The mergence of the two currents produces an interior sound, "Om."

Anahata Chakra The spiritual heart center.

Angaraka The planet Mars.

Arkaya The eleventh name of the Sun among the twelve names or powers of the Sun.

Ashwini Devatas A class of healing devas or angels.

Astrology The science of effects of vibration produced by the Sun, planets, and other heavenly bodies upon human beings and human affairs. The Eastern approach to this ancient science is lunar-based, and the Western approach is solar-based.

Atman The divine flame burning in the Hrit Padma, that goes by many names.

Avatar A divine being with no karma whatsoever who comes to Earth to perform specific beneficial tasks for humanity. There are many varieties and types of avatars.

Avish-vasa   Mistrust or general suspiciousness.

Bhanu   The fourth name of the Sun among the twelve names or powers of the Sun.

Bhaskara   The twelfth name of the Sun among the twelve names or powers of the Sun.

Bhaya   Fear.

Bija Mantra   A seed sound that contains spiritual power that must be grown or unwrapped through its repetition, frequently as part of a longer mantra.

Bodhisattva Vow   Buddhist oath to serve the development of sentient (conscious and self-aware) beings everywhere. A natural combination of compassion and the spirit of service.

Brahma   Personified Vedic God representative of the universe and all of its contents.

Brahma-Rishi   A sage (rishi) who has reached one of the highest possible states of knowledge while still an individual being. Reaching this state is possible only through a combination of effort and grace.

Brahmins   The Priest class and highest caste in India.

Budha   The planet Mercury.

Caduceus   The common medical symbol showing two serpents twining around a central staff, with wings sprouting at the top of the staff where the serpents meet. Also called the Staff of Hermes.

Chakra   Literally, "wheel" in Sanskrit. However, its common meaning refers to various spiritual centers located in the subtle body. Although there are dozens of chakras in the subtle body, the six located along the spine and the seventh at the top of the head are most commonly discussed.

Chandra   The Moon.

Cosmic Consciousness   Term for a state of consciousness, also called self-realization, where the essential unity of the universe is both perceived and understood.

Dambha   Arrogance.

Deva Lingua   Divine language, referring to Sanskrit.

Dhanvantre   The Celestial Physician.

Dharma   Divine Law.

Dum   Seed sound for Durga, the feminine power of protection.

Durga   Personified feminine power of protection.

Eim   Seed sound for Saraswati, the personified feminine power of knowledge, music, and sacred sound.

Gana   Power in one context; group in another context.

Ganesha (also called Ganapathi)   The personified power of unity that removes obstacles and assigns order to various spiritual powers and abilities.

Gayatri Mantra   The mantra often called "The Essence of the Vedas." This mantra on universal spiritual light and sound is practiced by Hindus of every caste and some branches of Buddhism who work with mantra.

Glaum   An additional seed sound for Ganesha that works powerfully in removing blocks between the genital center and the throat.

Grihna   Aversion or general disgust.

Guha   Divine personage who incarnated with the Avatar Rama and played the role of the ferry boatman. His meeting with Rama produced the blessing whereby the power of Rama's name would remove karma and lead to liberation.

Gum   Seed sound for Ganesha, also called Ganapathi, the power of unity that removes obstacles and assigns order to various spiritual powers and abilities.

Gurave   The planet Jupiter.

Guru   An enlightened spiritual teacher with the ability to transmit spiritual energy by one or more methods.

Hanuman   Monkey chieftain who became the foremost servant of the Avatar Rama.

Haum   Seed sound for Shiva, personification of universal consciousness.

Hinduism   The world's oldest religion with origins in India, stretching back for at least five thousand years according to some sources, and much longer according to others.

Hiranyagarbha   The seventh name of the Sun among the twelve names or powers of the Sun.

Hrim   Seed sound for the Hrit Padma.

Hrit Padma   An esoteric chakra located just below the heart center, often called the Sacred Heart.

Hum   Seed sound for the Vishuddha chakra located at the throat center of the subtle body.

I Ching   Chinese oracle-in-a-book, this spiritual tool can serve both as a source of spiritual learning and practical guidance.

Ida   The masculine current in the subtle body. One of the serpents shown in the Caduceus.

Incarnation   Individual life in a body. One is said to have many incarnations during the trek toward spiritual liberation at which time no more karma remains to be worked out.

Irsha   Jealousy.

Jagadamba   A term for "The World Mother." Any feminine person or archetype can be referred to as jagadamba. In Christianity, for instance, Mary is a jagadamba.

Jagadguru   An enlightened world teacher. Those spiritual figures around whom the world's great religions have formed are examples of jagadgurus.

Jaya   Victory.

Jnana   Spiritual knowledge.

Kalachakra   Literally, the "Wheel of Time." The Kalachakra deity of Tibetan Buddhism is a concrete symbol for the interplay of time, represented by a conjoining of masculine and feminine beings or parts of the same being. This masculine-feminine joining is called yub-yum in Tibetan Buddhism.

Kama   Desire. Also means unhealthy lust in certain situations.

Kapata-Ta   Duplicity, intentional deception.

Karma   The Law of Cause and Effect. The sum total of actions and thoughts that cause a reaction or return of like energy. Reincarnation or rebirth continues until all karma is balanced or neutralized.

Agami Karma   Returning karma from this and other lifetimes.

Kriyamana Karma   Immediate results from present actions.

Prarabdha Karma   Planetary karma represented by the natal birth chart as a particular birth or incarnation.

Sanchita Karma   Total of all karma from all lifetimes.

Ketu   The south karmic node (pole) of the Moon.

Khaga   The fifth name of the Sun among the twelve names or powers of the Sun.

Kheda   Paralyzing dejection.

Klim   Seed sound for attraction.

Krim   Seed sound for Kali, the feminine energy of destruction of negative ego.

Krodha   Anger.

Ksraum   Seed sound for Narasimha, the Man-Lion Avatar of Vishnu.

Kubera   Ancient spiritual being whose spiritual disciplines lead him to a position of supremacy over wealth.

Kundalini   The great feminine energy storehouse sitting coiled at the base of the spine. Awakening this energy and promoting its movement up the spine is the essence of spiritual progress.

Laja   Shame.

Lakshmana   Rama's younger brother who traveled with him when Rama was banished to the forest for twelve years.

Lakshmi   Personified feminine energy for wealth and abundance of all kinds.

Lam   Seed sound for the first chakra located at the base of the spine.

Lobha   Covetousness.

Loka A plane or level of existence. There are said to be seven upper luminous lokas, only three of which are physical in existence, and seven dark or nether lokas. Spiritual beings occupy the luminous lokas, while negative spirits inhabit the lower lokas. The Earth is said to be the first or bottom of the upper spheres of light. Thus, negative spirits are constantly trying to get here, where they can cause havoc.

Ma Sound resonating in the feminine or lunar current on the left side of the body, charging the pingala.

Mada Obstructing pride.

Maha Great. Also a plane (Maha Loka) in the nonphysical universe where sages and saints of high attainment are said to dwell.

Mahamaya The great illusion of this reality.

Maha Mrityunjaya Mantra The great mantra to defeat death and disease. Markandeya is the seer of this mantra.

Maha Rishi Great Sage.

Mah-Na Anger that is confined between two people.

Mala Rosary.

Manipura Chakra The third chakra located at the solar plexus.

Manjushri Personified Tibetan archetype or being who carries the sword of discriminitive reason.

Mantra Sanskrit spiritual formula.

Mantra Siddhi The power one attains when one has unwrapped the power of the mantra through repetition.

Marichi The eighth name of the Sun among the twelve names or powers of the Sun.

Markandeya A sixteen-year-old sage who was liberated from the necessity of rebirth by a cry to Shiva that subsequently became known as the Maha Mrityunjaya Mantra. Markandeya is the seer of this mantra practiced to combat disease and death.

Mata Mother.

Matsarya Envy.

Meru Bead The "head bead" on the mala or rosary. It is said that the power of repetition on the rosary comes to be stored here.

Mitra   The first name of the Sun among the twelve names or powers of the Sun.

Moha   Unhealthy attachment.

Mudra   Divine gesture. Exact placement of arms, hands, and fingers are said to produce specific energy effects if practiced by an Adept or spiritually advanced individual.

Muladhara Chakra   The first chakra located at the base of the spine.

Nada Brahma   The sound of the universe.

Nadis   Astral nerve tubes, similar to veins, that run through the subtle body.

Namaha   "Salutations," or "I salute." There are several words for this idea. This term has a neutral ending. See also "Swaha."

Narasimha   Man-Lion Avatar of Vishnu.

Narayana   Personification of the source of all this reality, including Brahma. Also, and concurrently, the threefold flame burning in the Hrit Padma. This seeming duality is intended to demonstrate that we may seem parted but are never really separated from God or the Divine.

Novena   Roman Catholic prayer discipline that usually runs for nine days, but sometimes runs for varying lengths for special purposes.

Om   Seed sound for the sixth chakra located at the brow center in the subtle body. Also, the sound heard when the masculine and feminine currents, Ida and Pingala, meet and merge at this location.

Parameshwari   The Supreme Feminine.

Pingala   Feminine energy channel in the subtle body. One of the serpents shown in the Caduceus.

Pishu-Nata   Fickleness.

Prajapathi   "Forefathers" of the human race. These luminous beings aided in the process of adding divinity to the human race by contributing some of their own essence so many eons ago that it is uncertain just where this idea came from.

Prana   Life energy that fills the human body. There are five types.

Prana   The energy that circulates in the body. It can be transferred from individual to individual, as healers often do.

Samana   The energy that exists uniformly throughout the body and distributes energy from digested food.

Udana   The energy that separates the consciousness from the body during sleep.

Upana   The eliminating energy that governs processing out of waste material and energy from the body.

Vyana   The energy that provides the sense of touch.

Puja   Ceremonial worship.

Purusha   Transcendental overself. The aggregate spiritual soul-mind of humanity and yet more as well.

Pushne   Sanskrit designation for the sixth name of the Sun among the twelve names or powers of the Sun.

Ra   Sound that invokes energy in the Ida or masculine energy channel in the subtle body.

Rahu   The north karmic node of the Moon.

Ram   Seed sound for the third chakra located at the solar plexus.

Rama   Avatar of Vishnu.

Ravi   The second name of the Sun among the twelve names or powers of the Sun.

Rudraksha   A berry found in northern India that, when dried and hardened, is drilled and strung to form a prayer necklace (rosary) called a "mala." This berry is said to be especially useful in holding energy relating to Shiva and Durga (Kali).

Sadhana   Regular spiritual discipline.

Sage   A person or being with tangible spiritual knowledge.

Sam-Brahma   General state of constant agitation.

Samsara   The "ocean of rebirth" that the soul must traverse until it reaches the shores of liberation from such rebirth.

Sandhya The meeting of the day and the night. Dusk and dawn are said to be spiritually potent times every day. Many traditional spiritual teachers from the East will instruct their students to perform their disciplines at these times.

Sanskrit A language no longer spoken by any nation or group, but still widely used in the religions of Hinduism and Buddhism. The alphabet of this language is said to be inscribed upon the petals of the chakras, giving it the title of "Language of the chakras," "Language of the gods," or the "Divine language."

Saraswati Personified feminine energy for the arts, sciences, spiritual pursuits, and knowledge of all kinds.

Sat Truth. Also called "Satyam."

Saturn Return (also called the "Saturn Period") The time when the planet Saturn returns to the exact point it occupied at the moment of one's birth. The "return" is said to trigger a new 28.9-year learning cycle. This time period is the period of Saturn's revolution around the Sun. Most people have two Saturn returns in a lifetime, at approximately ages twenty-nine and fifty-nine.

Savitre The tenth name of the Sun among the twelve names or powers of the Sun.

Seer A sage who has discovered a mantra or spiritual concept not previously known.

Self-Realization A state of consciousness where the essential unity of the universe is both perceived and understood. This state is also called cosmic consciousness.

Shabda Brahma The sacred sound of the universe, also known as Nada Brahma.

Shaivism The study of consciousness and its attributes through Shiva, commonly known as the masculine principle in the universe.

Shakti A generic term for feminine power or energy. See "Kundalini."

Shani The planet Saturn.

Shanti A dynamic state of peace.

Shiva A personification of consciousness, said to be male.

Shoka Grief.

Shrim   Seed sound for Lakshmi, the feminine energy of abundance.

Shukra   Sanskrit designation for the planet Venus.

Shu-Shupti   Laziness.

Siddha   One who has attained siddhi.

Siddhi   Power or spiritual ability.

Sikhism   A world religion that is a fusion of Hinduism and Islam. Male practitioners of this religion usually wear turbans and let their hair and beards grow.

Subramanya   Eldest son of Shiva in the Hindu Pantheon. Also goes by Kartikeya and Skanda.

Subtle Body   An energy body that interpenetrates and interacts with the physical body. It is here that the chakras are found.

Suktam   Hymn, usually to a specific deity, such as the Narayana Suktam or the Purusha Suktam.

Surya   The third name of the Sun among the twelve names or powers of the Sun.

Swadhisthana Chakra   The second chakra, located at the genital center.

Swaha   Another term for "I salute" or "I offer." This term has a feminine ending. See also "Namaha."

Tantra   The joining of masculine and feminine energy for a particular purpose. This term is one of the most confusing in the Eastern lexicon. At its essence, it means working with the energy of nature or the energy available in the universe at large. One accessible route to this energy is through the power inherent in women. Tantric rites in ancient Hindu temples strove to give the power inherent in women to the priests via ritual sexual activities.

Tara   Tibetan Universal Mother.

Upaguru   The omnipresent "teacher without form" that can manifest in seemingly bizarre ways. It can appear as "the magazine article that seems like it was written just for you," or "a statement by an actor in a televised drama that is so powerful for you that it nearly brings you out of your chair." These are examples of how the up-aguru may teach and lead. It is a principle residing in everyone.

Upanishads Sacred texts summarized over several thousand years. What exists today is only a remnant of what once existed.

Vajra Thunderbolt. Used predominantly in Tibetan spiritual constructs.

Vajrapani The Great Initiator. With both a beautiful and horrific visage, Vajrapani is often depicted holding a thunderbolt aloft, symbolic of his great power. As the Tibetan protector, he drives away demonic influences. As the Great Initiator, he reveals the mysteries of spiritual practice to the sincere initiate.

Vajrasattva The Great Purifier. Chanting of the 100-syllabled Tibetan mantra is a staple of Buddhist practices. The visualization practice that accompanies it shows black gunk flowing from the body into the Earth where the negative energy can be processed and recycled.

Vam Seed sound for the second chakra located at the genital center.

Vasanas Emotional and mental tendencies stored in the subconscious mind.

Vasistha One of seven Brahma-rishis who are said to be with humanity from one great cycle to the next, helping and guiding the spiritual development of the species.

Vasudeva The "Indweller" in everyone. Another name for the flame in the Hrit Padma. Also the name of Krishna's father in the *Mahabharata*.

Vedas Four central scriptures from the Upanishads that were never summarized and remain intact. They are the Rig Veda, Sama Veda, Yajur Veda, and Artharva Veda.

Vishada Incapacitating sadness.

Vishnu The Vedic God of Preservation. It is said that all true spiritual leaders and teachers from any religion carry the energy of Vishnu.

Vishuddha Chakra The fifth chakra located at the throat center.

Vishwamitra   A Brahma-rishi who attained this status by arduous
   spiritual practice and a final stamp of divine grace from Brahma-
   rishi Vasistha. When that moment occurred, Vishwamitra experienced the Gayatri mantra, becoming its seer.

Yajna   Sacrifice, usually in the sense of a ritual fire worship ceremony in which negative karma can be consumed.
Yam   Seed sound for the fourth chakra located at the heart center in
   the subtle body.

Bibliography

Andrews, Ted. *Music Therapy for Non-Musicians*. Batavia, Ohio: Dragonhawk Publishing, 1997.

Arnold, Sir Edwin, trans. *The Song Celestial or Bhagavad-gita*. 1885; Los Angeles: Self-Realization Fellowship, 1977.

Ashley-Farrand, Thomas. *The Ancient Science of Sanskrit Mantra and Ceremony;* vol. I, *Mantra,* and vol. 2, *Great Spiritual Disciplines and Ceremonies*. Privately published, 1996; available at www.sanskritmantra.com.

————. *True Stories of Spiritual Power*. Privately published, 1995; available at www.sanskritmantra.com.

Avalon, Arthur [pseud. of Sir John Woodroffe], trans. *Tantra of the Great Liberation*. 1913; New York: Dover Publications, 1972.

Basso, Keith H. *The Cibecue Apache*. Case Studies in Cultural Anthropology. New York: Holt, Rinehart & Winston, 1910; 1970.

Berendt, Joachim-Ernst. *Nada Brahma: The World Is Sound: Music and the Landscape of Consciousness*. Rochester, Vt.: Destiny Books, 1987.

Bernbaum, Edwin. *The Way to Shambhala*. Los Angeles: Jeremy P. Tarcher, 1980.

Beyer, Stephen. *The Cult of Tara: Magic and Ritual in Tibet*. Berkeley: University of California Press, 1973.

Blavatsky, H. P. *The Secret Doctrine*. 1888; Pasadena, Calif.: Theosophical University Press, 1970.

Blofeld, John. *Mantras: Sacred Words of Power*. New York: E. P. Dutton, 1977.

Board of Scholars. *Mantramahoddadhi*. Delhi, India: Sri Satguru Publications, 1984.

Chawdhri, L. R. *Practicals of Mantra & Tantra*. New Delhi, India: Sagar Publications, 1990.

Dalai Lama XIV [Tenzin Gyatso]. *The Kalachakra Tantra: Rite of Initiation for the Stage of Generation.* Boston: Wisdom Publications, 1985.

Danielou, Alain. *The Gods of India: Hindu Polytheism.* New York: Inner Traditions International, 1985.

Elkin, A. P. *The Australian Aborigines.* 5th ed. Garden City, N.Y.: Anchor Books, 1974.

Epstein, Pearle. *Kabbalah: The Way of the Jewish Mystic.* Garden City, N.Y.: Doubleday, 1978.

Guthrie, Kenneth Sylvan, comp. and trans. *The Pythagorean Sourcebook and Library: An Anthology of Ancient Writings Which Relate to Pythagoras and Pythagorean Philosophy.* Grand Rapids, Mich.: Phanes Press, 1987.

Harshananda, Swami. *Hindu Gods and Goddesses.* Mysore, India: Sri Ramakrishna Ashrama, 1982.

Le Mée, Katherine. *Chant.* New York: Bell Tower, 1994.

Li Jicheng and Ku Shoukang (text) and Kang Song (photos). *The Realm of Tibetan Buddhism.* Edited by Xisao Shiling and An Chunyang. Translated by Wang Weijiong. San Francisco: China Books & Periodicals, 1985.

Malinowski, Bronislaw. *Argonauts of the Western Pacific: An Account of Native Enterprise and Adventure in the Archipelagoes of Melanesian New Guinea.* New York: E. P. Dutton, 1922; 1961.

Mayo, Jeff. *The Planets and Human Behavior.* Reno, Nev.: CRCS Publications, 1972.

Sivananda, Swami, trans. and comm. *The Bhagavad Gita.* Durban, South Africa: Sivananda Press, 1972.

———. *Japa Yoga: A Comprehensive Treatise on Mantra-shastra.* Sivanandanagar: Divine Life Society, 1972.

Tompkins, Peter, and Christopher Bird. *The Secret Life of Plants.* New York: Harper & Row, 1973.

Turnbull, Colin. *Wayward Servants: The Two Worlds of the African Pygmies.* New York: Simon & Schuster, 1962.

Yogananda, Paramahansa. *Autobiography of a Yogi.* 1946; Los Angeles: Self-Realization Fellowship, 1995.

Zajonc, R. B. "Feeling and Thinking." *American Psychologist,* February 1980.

INTERNET RESOURCES

www.hubcom.com/tantric/frtan.htm
www.mozarteffect.com

Index

About the Author

THOMAS ASHLEY-FARRAND (Namadeva) practiced mantra-based spiritual disciplines since 1973 and was an acknowledged expert in Sanskrit mantra spiritual disciplines. Vedic Priest, author, and international lecturer and storyteller, Mr. Ashley-Farrand made presentations in the U.S. and Canada as well as India. He was priest-in-residence for the Temple of Cosmic Religion in Washington, D.C., from 1973 to 1980. Thomas lived in Southern California, with his wife, Satyabhama, an attorney in private practice, who often performed the ancient Vedic ceremonies with him. He died in 2010.

www.sanskritmantra.com.